ARTHRITIS

OTHER BOOKS BY JAMES F. FRIES, M.D.

The Arthritis Helpbook
by Kate Lorig and James F. Fries

Living Well
by James F. Fries

Take Care of Yourself
by Donald M. Vickery and James F. Fries

Taking Care of Your Child
by Robert H. Pantell, James F. Fries, and Donald M. Vickery

Vitality and Aging
by James F. Fries and Lawrence M. Crapo

CONTENTS

PREFACE

Arthritis can be defeated. Not easily and not always—but usually and substantially. Recently there has been an explosion in scientific knowledge about arthritis. Dramatic new treatments are available. Your doctor can help more than ever before. But *you* need to be in charge of your health. This book will guide you toward working effectively with your doctor and toward your personal plan of action. You need to think in terms of self-management rather than just self-care. You need to manage your medical treatment and the use of your own resources. All of the latest information is in this book, and you need to use it.

Four principles provide the intellectual framework for this book. In the first edition two decades ago, these thoughts were new, but the success of programs based on these principles has established them as the foundation of sound arthritis self-management.

First, it is crucial that each individual assume greater personal responsibility for his or her own health, and that dependable information sources are available—the medical consumer has a right to know the facts.

Second, a revolution in medical thinking has occurred; it is now known that the body lasts longer when it is used and ages more rapidly with disuse. This concept has been emphasized for cardiac and muscular fitness; it also holds to a surprising degree for strengthening the joints. For example, long-distance runners do *not* frequently get arthritis.

Third, withdrawal from social interaction, from new experiences, and from the exercise of personal autonomy all accelerate the aging process. Arthritis is in many ways a physical parallel to aging; it is an allegory for the aging process. When arthritis is incorrectly considered an inevitable problem of increasing pain and decreasing function, it becomes a reason to retreat from independent life. Treatment of arthritis thus extends far beyond the joints. The successful response to musculoskeletal pain must be reaffirmation of life rather than its rejection.

Fourth, if you think you can do it, you can do it. For some people arthritis teaches frustration and helplessness; these people don't do very well. For others, who maintain the belief that their actions can change their future, arthritis has relatively little effect on their lives.

In this edition I have highlighted the revolution in doctors' treatment strategy for rheumatoid arthritis, and I have indicated the role of exciting new medications. I have stressed the important relationship between lack of exercise and the development of disability from arthritis. In our companion volume, *The Arthritis Helpbook,* Dr. Kate Lorig and I provide additional practical details for implementing your own program for success in dealing with your arthritis. The self-management techniques developed for *Take Care of Yourself* and used in *Taking Care of Your Child* and *Living Well* are employed again in this volume. I hope that they succeed in clarifying this neglected and critically important disease area.

J.F.F.

Stanford, California
May 1999

ACKNOWLEDGMENTS

Among those to whom I am indebted for my understanding of the concepts of arthritis self-management are: Margaret Baltes, Paul Baltes, James Birren, Kenneth Brandt, John Bunker, Lionel Cosin, Lawrence Crapo, René Dubos, Alain Enthoven, Jack Farquhar, Victor Fuchs, Halsted Holman, John Knowles, Kate Lorig, Ralph Paffenbarger, Matilda Riley, David Rogers, Martin Seligman, and Anne Somers.

I am also indebted to the many patients, physicians, and patient educators who contributed experiences and perspective to the development of this manuscript. Their suggestions have resulted in hundreds of specific additions and changes. Remaining deficiencies are my responsibility.

I particularly acknowledge the contributions of:

The Arthritis Foundation, Dr. Jack Boyer, Dr. Melvin Britton, Dr. Stephen Coles, Dr. George Ehrlich, Dr. Wallace Epstein, Lois Fleming, Dr. Bevra Hahn, Dr. Evelyn Hess, Dr. L. A. Healey, Dr. Marc Hochberg, Dr. Michael Lockshin, Kate Lorig, R.N., Dr.P.H., Dr. Dennis McShane, Dena Ramey, Dr. John Miller III, Dr. Donald Mitchell, Janice Pigg, R.N., Irene Seligman, Patricia Spitz, R.N., Dr. Robert Swezey, Annette Swezey, M.P.H., Dr. Cody Wasner, and Dr. Gordon Williams. Special thanks are due to the editorial staff at Perseus Books.

HOW TO USE THIS BOOK

This book can be a great help to you if used correctly. More arthritis information is provided here than has previously been publicly available. This book will help you understand your arthritis and your doctor's treatments, and it may provide you with more detailed explanations than your doctor has time to give. The medical content of this book has been reviewed by many physicians expert in the care of patients with arthritis. I indicate consensus on a particular point by using *we;* if my opinion might differ from those of some of my colleagues, I have used *I* to indicate the source.

But this book is not a doctor. All serious forms of arthritis require the care of a physician. In an individual case, the recommendations given in this book may not be just right. So if you are under the care of a physician and receive advice contrary to this book, follow the physician's advice. This ensures that the individual characteristics of your case are taken into account.

There are many different kinds of arthritis, but you will usually be bothered by only one. There are many drugs that may be useful, many tests that may be performed, and many surgical operations that may be appropriate. You will need only a few. This book is organized to guide you to the sections that pertain to you, letting you skip over those that do not apply.

Read what you need now. Next month or next year you may need to refer to different sections.

There are three important steps that you can take toward defeating your arthritis, and this book is organized around them:

- Part I of this book will help you **identify what kind of arthritis you have** and choose the best treatment approach to defeat it. Use the simple charts in Chapter 2 to identify your category of arthritis. Each of the next eight chapters includes a detailed discussion on a specific type of arthritis. These discussions provide pertinent information on the best treatment, medication, and tests for your type of arthritis.

- Part II has important information on **managing your arthritis,** including: treatments (Chapter 13), medications (Chapters 14, 15, and 16), surgery (Chapter 17), tests (Chapter 18), avoiding quack treatments (Chapter 19), saving money (Chapter 20), and preventing arthritis (Chapter 21).
- Part III is designed to help you **manage your everyday problems** with pain, medication side effects, getting around, sexual relations, and work. Look up your specific problems in the table of contents. Read the appropriate sections and use the charts in these sections to help you decide whether you can treat yourself at home or need to see a doctor or other health professional.

PART I

Understanding Your Arthritis

CHAPTER 1

Defeating Arthritis

You have much more control over your arthritis or rheumatism than you may think. You do not have to be a victim. Rather, you can defeat these problems and lead a full, satisfying life. To do this, you need to know something about arthritis. You need to know how to prevent damage to joint tissues. And you need to know what is happening in your body and what you can do about it. You need to become an **arthritis self-manager.**

For some curious reason, the idea lingers that "nothing can be done for arthritis." The very opposite is true. Probably more progress has been made in the fight against arthritis than in the struggle against our other major diseases—cancer, heart disease, and diabetes. You can benefit from these advances.

The battle against certain forms of arthritis is nearly won. Rheumatoid arthritis, the most common major arthritis, is under attack from a number of exciting new treatments. Gout, a major disease in the past, now yields readily to treatment. Systemic lupus erythematosus, once a mysterious and very serious ailment, is now successfully managed in almost every case. Ankylosing spondylitis no longer leads to severe deformity except in the most unusual cases. Surgical advances, such as joint replacement, often prove dramatically helpful. Genetic factors have been identified for many kinds of arthritis, and our understanding of the molecular basis for joint disease is increasing rapidly.

As arthritis has become better understood, its complexity has become more apparent. Over one hundred different kinds of arthritis have now been identified. Every kind of arthritis, and ultimately every patient, is different. For treatment to be effective, it is essential to find the treatment most appropriate for the individual patient. Knowledge of how to match treatment to patient accurately is not yet complete, and many patients have to undergo several kinds of treatment before the right one is found. If you know about recent advances in the field and the problems yet to be solved, you can help with your own treatment program.

Successfully managing your arthritis depends as much on you as on your doctor. Your decisions are ultimately the most important. You decide:

- How much activity to undertake
- Whether to see the doctor, and when
- What kind of doctor to see
- When to ask for a second opinion
- Whether to accept the medical advice offered
- Whether to follow a treatment program carefully
- Whether to seek a quack treatment or to believe a sensational claim of a miracle cure

Ultimately, you decide how much you exercise, what you think of yourself, and what you want to do with your life. Your doctor can be a great help to you. But you have to make the decisions and carry them out.

Think of this book as a series of conversations with your doctor about your problems. We who treat patients with arthritis have had these conversations hundreds of times. But sometimes the demands of office or clinic don't give us enough time for in-depth discussions with individual patients. Sometimes information from a discussion is forgotten by the patient, or only part of it is remembered. Often the patient thinks of new questions after the visit is over. Here you can read and reread the discussion in full, and you can refer to pertinent sections to refresh your understanding when a particular problem arises.

An "arthritis victim" is someone who has been defeated by arthritis. Your goal is to defeat your arthritis—to come out on top. Your arthritis can be helped; in some cases, it can be cured. Even when it cannot be cured, your life can be full and complete. You can be independent and happy. This book is about resources: medical resources, community resources, and, most important, your own resources. This book is about how to defeat the pains and stiffness in your body.

If You Have Pain, Do You Have Arthritis?

In the truest sense of the word, most "arthritis" is not really arthritis at all! Doctors use the term **arthritis** differently from patients. The *arth* part of the word means "joint"—not muscle, tendon, ligament, or bone. The *itis* part means "inflamed." Thus, true arthritis affects the joints, and the affected joints are inflamed—red, warm, swollen, or tender when squeezed. If you do not have any of these symptoms, then you do not have arthritis in the true sense of the term.

However, in common usage and in this book, the term *arthritis* refers to almost any painful condition of the muscles or the skeletal system. **Rheumatism** is an imprecise term that includes not only problems with the joints, but any problems affecting the body's musculoskeletal system. In this book we have taken a very broad view of what constitutes arthritis and rheumatism, and you will find descriptions and treatments for all major problems affecting the muscles, joints, and the areas around the joints—from rheumatoid arthritis to fibromyalgia to sciatica to bursitis.

How Common Is Arthritis?

In the United States, over 75 million people experience some symptoms in their joints and muscles from time to time. Twenty-two million have moderate problems from their arthritis, and nearly 3 million Americans are severely affected. Thus, we can talk about arthritis either as a national problem that, although very common, is usually relatively mild, or as an extremely severe problem that affects a relatively small number of people. Whichever way you look at it, arthritis and rheumatism cause more work loss, more pain, and more poor functioning in daily life than any other kind of human illness. But arthritis can be prevented in many cases, and effective treatment is available for all forms of these diseases.

Do You Need a Doctor?

Few of us go even a single year without some episode of pain or stiffness. So we have to be able to decide when a condition requires a physician's care and when we can take care of it ourselves. The decision chart presented on the next page will help you answer this general question. If you have one of the specific problems listed in Part III, "Solving Problems with Arthritis," refer to that particular decision chart for assistance in deciding whether to see the doctor.

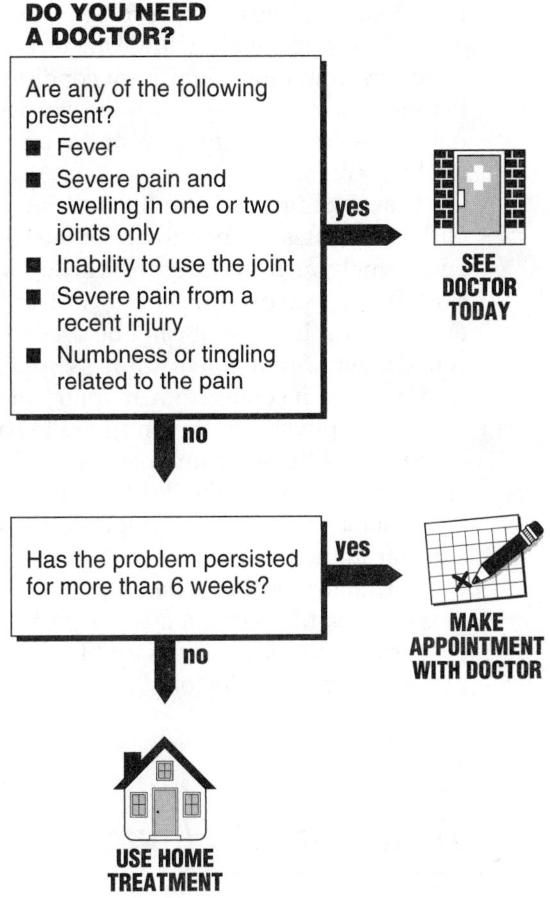

Only rarely does a patient with muscle or joint pain need a physician immediately. Home treatment and patience will resolve most problems. It is important to remember that, for most problems involving the musculoskeletal system, the natural healing process requires two to six weeks. Drugs do not accelerate this natural healing process. For most common problems, therefore, a period of watchful waiting is the most important treatment.

The relative emergencies are infection, nerve damage, fractures near a joint, and gout. In the first three, serious damage may result if the joint is neglected; in the fourth, the pain is so intense that immediate help is needed. *Immediate* means to call or see a doctor today. Most complications of arthritis occur slowly and are more easily prevented than corrected. A persistent musculoskeletal problem always should be brought to the attention of a physician, but allow "tincture of time" to sort out trivial injuries or strains from more significant conditions. Remember that arthritis results in more lost work days and more sickness than any other kind of disease; it must be managed correctly and with care. Not too much concern, but not too little either.

Run your finger down the decision chart. Fever, usually over 100°F (38°C), indicates the possibility of infection or a severe form of arthritis. Surprisingly, arthritis affecting only a few joints is more urgent than arthritis affecting many joints. Both gout and infection usually involve only one or two joints. If the joint can't be used, it may be significantly injured and it is in danger of permanent stiffness. Again, immediate attention is required. And if the pain comes from an injury that might have caused a broken bone, see a physician. If pain from the back runs down the side of the leg to the foot, if there is numbness or tingling in the fingers, or if there is an area of numbness on the head when you move your neck, there may be nerve damage. Any such symptoms should be brought to the attention of a doctor immediately.

Fortunately arthritis pains aren't very often associated with any of those things. More frequently the problem will simply go away slowly over several weeks. When a problem persists for more than six weeks, it is wise to consult a doctor.

Treatment at Home

If you are going to wait six weeks, what can you do at home? Rest, warmth, and minor pain medication make up the initial home treatment. Remember that the purpose of pain is not to make us miserable but to prevent us from injuring ourselves further. If a joint is painful when you move it, your body is telling you to rest that part. Using too much pain medication can mask the body's pain message and result in overuse of an inflamed joint. This can cause additional damage. So keep the pain relief mild and simple. The following dosages are often satisfactory for adults: aspirin, two tablets four times a day; acetaminophen (Tylenol) in the same dosage; ibuprofen (Advil, Nuprin), one tablet four times a day; or naproxen (Aleve), one tablet two times a day.

What else can you do for yourself? There are hundreds of other measures you can take. Read about them in the remainder of Part I and in Part II, and under the headings of your particular problems in Part III.

Time is the only known cure for most problems that affect the musculoskeletal system. When you develop a new complaint, you must use time to separate the trivial from the serious. Luckily the trivial outnumber the serious by at least 20 to 1. In most instances the body's repair process involves resting the affected part and bringing in new protein and fibrous materials with which to reconstruct the injured area. Through most of this book we will be focusing on the small percentage of musculoskeletal problems that time alone will not cure, problems that may result in significant health difficulties.

CHAPTER 2

What Kind of Arthritis Do You Have?

There are 127 kinds of arthritis currently known. They range from rare to common and from trivial to serious. Unfortunately, too many people think of arthritis as a single disease. Selecting the treatment that will help you the most depends on knowing the type of arthritis that is active in your body.

You can understand the process that is causing your pain or stiffness without reading about 127 diseases or going to medical school. Arthritis has only eight major categories, and this chapter differentiates them. Each of the next eight chapters describes one category in more detail. Chapter 11 discusses connective-tissue diseases that can resemble arthritis. Chapter 12 discusses osteoporosis. This "brittle bone" condition is not arthritis, but it can result in bone damage as crippling as the more severe forms of arthritis.

Some arthritis diagnoses can be difficult for even the most skilled physicians and may require laboratory tests and X-rays. Your doctor is more experienced than you are at making the observations that help in the diagnosis. Any person with arthritis who meets the criteria noted in Chapter 1 or who has pain for longer than six weeks should be seen by a physician. So be sure you have a doctor. You shouldn't deal with serious arthritis alone.

But you can help your doctor a great deal by understanding what is happening in your body and what can be done about it. Identify your arthritis category. This will help you better understand why you are experiencing certain symptoms. But leave the diagnosis to your doctor.

The diagram on page 9 shows a typical joint. The joint is faced with a layer of *cartilage* (or gristle) on each side. The joint membrane, called the *synovial membrane,* surrounds the joint space and provides lubricating fluid for the cartilage surfaces. Fibrous tissue (the *joint capsule*) connects the bones and gives stability to the joint. Muscles taper down into *tendons* and attach to the bone, usually just above or just below a joint. In some parts of

Where Arthritis Attacks

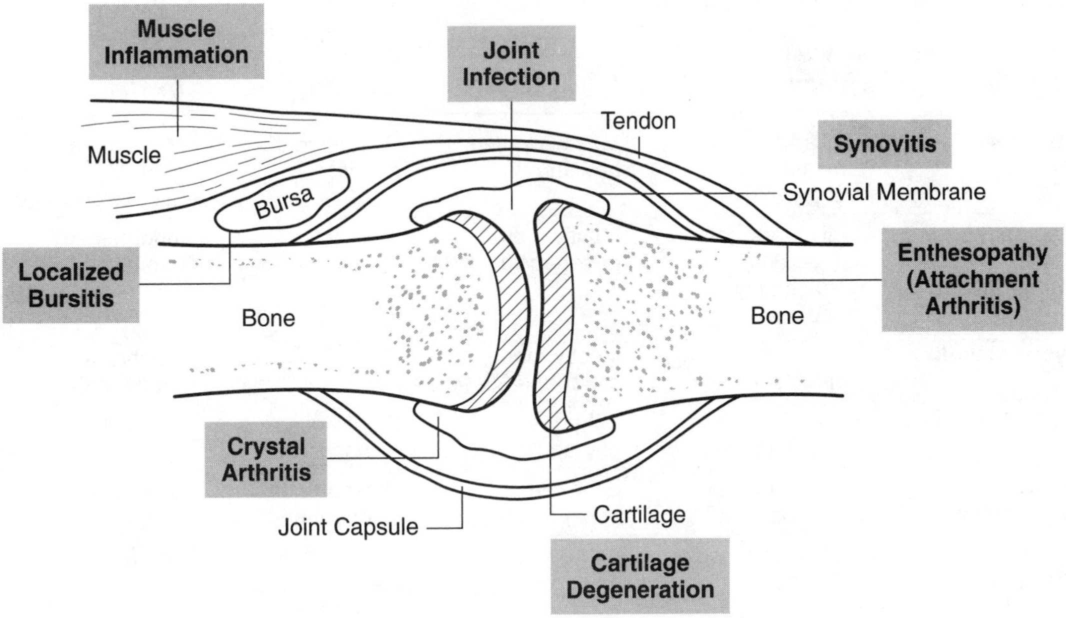

the body, *bursae* lie between two muscles (or between muscles and tendons) to lubricate body tissues that must move across each other.

That's the anatomy lesson. The joint is remarkably well engineered. The cartilage is spongy and absorbs shock, the joint is self-lubricating, and also self-healing following injury. Now that you know the anatomy, you're ready to understand the eight categories. Different categories of arthritis generally attack different body structures.

The Eight Major Categories

Table 2.1, "Arthritis Categories," summarizes the eight categories in a simple way. There are exceptions to these rules, but we will get to those later. Notice that each category has a different basic problem and a different basic treatment.

The first category is **synovitis.** This big word simply means that the synovial membrane, which creates the lubricating fluid for the joint, is

TABLE 2.1 *Arthritis Categories*

Category	*What's happening?*	*Who gets it?*	*Most typical diseases in this category*	*Typical treatment*
Synovitis	Inflamed membrane of the joint	Mostly women, any age	Rheumatoid arthritis	Methotrexate, gold, hydroxychloroquine
Attachment arthritis (enthesopathy)	Inflamed ligament or tendon attachment to bone	Mostly men, onset age 15–40	Ankylosing spondylitis	Indomethacin, naproxen
Crystal arthritis	Chemical crystals in the joint fluid	Mostly men, onset age 35–90	Gout	Colchicine, allopurinol
Joint infection	Bacteria in the joint fluid	Either sex, any age	*Staphylococcus, Gonococcus*	Antibiotics
Cartilage degeneration	Breakdown of joint cartilage	Either sex, onset age 45–90	Osteoarthrosis osteoarthritis	Low-dose aspirin
Muscle inflammation	Inflamed muscle tissues	Either sex, any age	Polymyalgia rheumatica, polymyositis	Prednisone
Local conditions	Local injury	Either sex, any age	Low back strain, tennis elbow, frozen shoulder	Local measures
General conditions	Poorly defined	Either sex, any age	Fibromyalgia	Exercise

inflamed. Inflammation makes it red, warm, tender, or swollen. The major disease with synovitis is called *rheumatoid arthritis,* or *RA.* It can occur at any age and it affects mostly women. Treatment is different for every individual, but typically effective treatments are hydroxychloroquine, methotrexate, leflunomide, and intramuscular gold, among others.

The second category I have named **attachment arthritis.** This term is a new one, and your doctor may not be familiar with it. I have used it to help you understand the process. Doctors often call this disease process *enthesopathy,* but people have trouble understanding this word. Here, the primary inflammation occurs not in the joint membrane but where the ligaments and tendons attach to the bone. This condition affects men more often than women and usually begins between age 15 and age 40. *Ankylosing spondylitis* (*AS* or "poker spine") is the most common attachment arthritis.

Crystal arthritis is sometimes called **microcrystalline arthritis** by physicians, because the crystals for which the condition is named are very small. These crystals form in the joint space itself. As the body tries to remove the crystals a painful inflammation occurs. The most dramatic example is *gout*. These conditions affect men more frequently than women and usually begin in middle life or later.

Joint infections make up the fourth category. Here there are bacteria or other germs in the joint fluid. These infections can occur at any age and in either sex; young persons are most frequently infected with the *Gonococcus* (GC) bacterium, while older individuals frequently have the *Staphylococcus* (staph) germ.

Cartilage degeneration is the fifth category. The cartilage that faces the joints can break down with age. As the cartilage splits and frays, the ends of the bones themselves may come in contact with each other. This forms the arthritis we call *osteoarthritis* or *osteoarthrosis.* It usually is noticed in middle life or later and is so common that all of us, if we live long enough, will experience some features of it. It is not really due to "wear and tear," but it does become more common with age.

The sixth category is **muscle inflammation.** This problem isn't really in the joint at all. Many patients complaining of arthritis actually have problems in the muscles or other tissues. These diseases are more unusual and can affect either sex at any age.

Local conditions make up the seventh category. For the most part, local problems result from local irritation or injury, not from disease. The back has suffered a strain or a sprain, there is pull of the ligament around the elbow as a result of playing tennis—this or some other minor accident, often unnoticed, has led to pain in a single region of the body. If you treat these conditions carefully they usually aren't much of a problem. These are the most common of all medical problems. They include low back pain, bursitis, tendinitis, frozen shoulder, and many other familiar syndromes.

The eighth category is termed **general conditions.** These conditions involve aching and stiffness throughout the body. They can occur in either sex and at any age, but they are rather more common in the thirties, forties, and early fifties than at other ages. Doctors are just beginning to recognize some of the different conditions within this group. *Fibromyalgia* is the most common general condition.

Identifying Your Arthritis Category

The decision chart on the next page will help you quickly determine your arthritis category. This chart will give you the correct category about 90% of the time, and if you double-check your result with Table 2.2, "Features of Arthritis Categories," on page 14 and with the discussion in the appropriate section of this chapter, you are unlikely to be misled. Your doctor will use a more complicated logic to determine the category of your arthritis, but this decision chart has been constructed using questions you can answer yourself. If your doctor has told you what your diagnosis is, look it up in the index, then go directly to the pertinent discussion.

Let's look at the reasons for the questions posed in the decision chart. How many parts of the body hurt? Infections, crystal arthritis, and local conditions usually affect only one part of the body, and synovitis and cartilage degeneration sometimes affect only one part. Distinction between these takes place as we move across the chart, responding to successive questions.

Is a single joint warm, swollen, or tender? Remember that pain in the muscles and joints is not the same as true arthritis, which by definition means "inflamed joint." If there is not true arthritis, then by definition we have a "local condition," such as an injury or tendinitis. Arthritis in a child (under 16) may be the synovitis of juvenile rheumatoid arthritis or acute rheumatic fever. If fever and a "single hot joint" are present in an adult, infection must be suspected. If the pain persists for over two weeks, cartilage degeneration in a single joint, perhaps a knee, is likely; rarely it may be a synovitis. The single hot joint without any fever or injury is likely to be a crystal arthritis.

Suppose that several parts of the body hurt. Then we use the left side of the decision chart. If low back pain or heel pain is present, the problem is likely to be an attachment arthritis. If the low back hasn't been affected, the question is whether there are obvious signs of inflammation in a joint. If so, then it is most likely a synovitis. If not, are there signs of inflammation in the muscles? If all answers are no, then it is most likely a general condition. Synovitis usually is associated with discomfort in the morning lasting 30 minutes or longer, while cartilage degeneration leads to more discomfort later in the day. Synovitis usually involves both sides of the body relatively equally, involves a different group of joints, and is more "boggy" to the touch over the joint, but these distinctions are often difficult to make, even for the doctor.

After you have determined a category, check Table 2.2, "Features of Arthritis Categories," on page 14 to see if the category makes sense for your arthritis. The severity of the inflammation is greatest with crystal

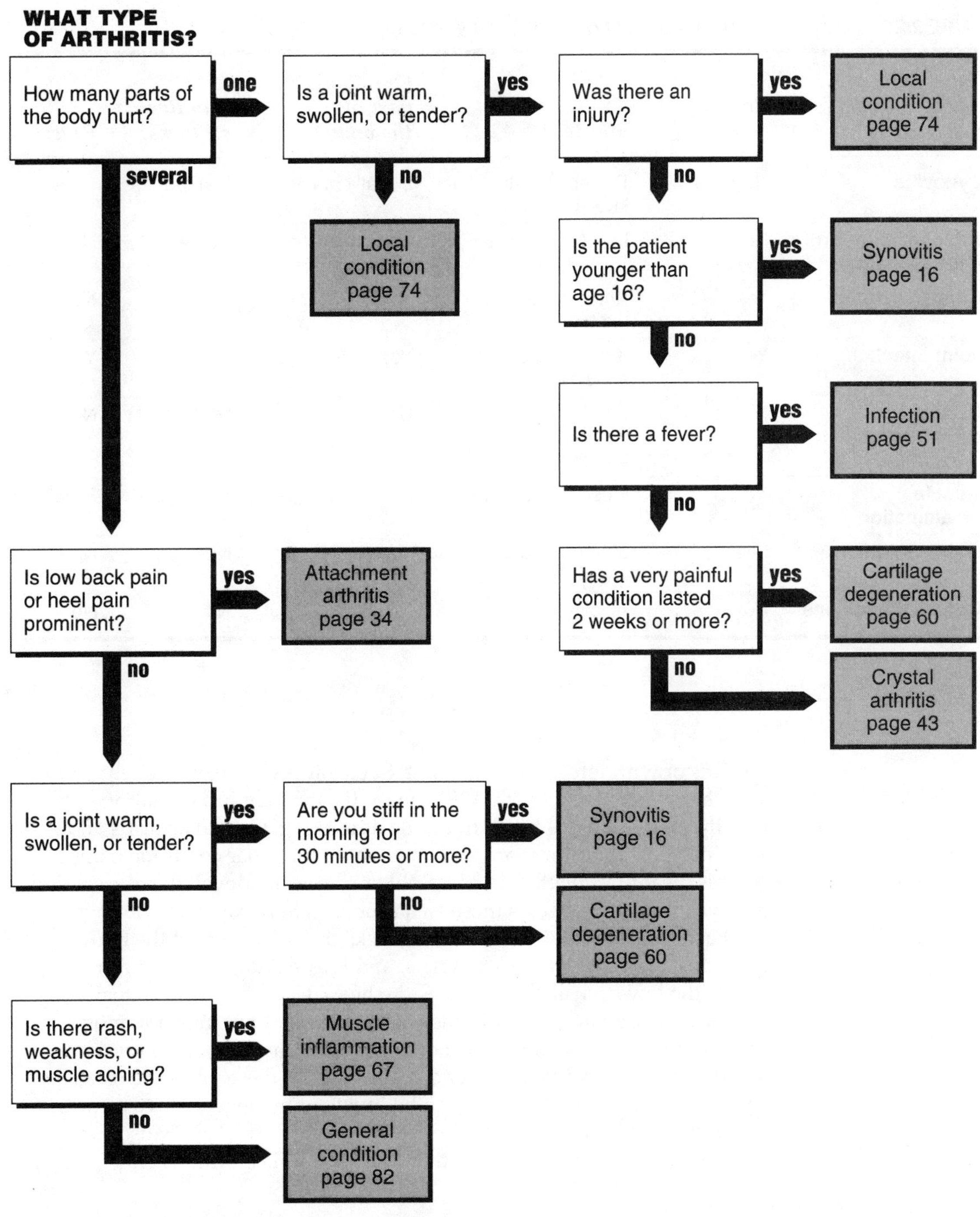
WHAT TYPE
OF ARTHRITIS?
How many parts of the body hurt?
one
several
Is a joint warm, swollen, or tender?
yes
no
Local condition page 74
Was there an injury?
yes
no
Local condition page 74
Is the patient younger than age 16?
yes
no
Synovitis page 16
Is there a fever?
yes
no
Infection page 51
Has a very painful condition lasted 2 weeks or more?
yes
no
Cartilage degeneration page 60
Crystal arthritis page 43
Is low back pain or heel pain prominent?
yes
no
Attachment arthritis page 34
Is a joint warm, swollen, or tender?
yes
no
Are you stiff in the morning for 30 minutes or more?
yes
no
Synovitis page 16
Cartilage degeneration page 60
Is there rash, weakness, or muscle aching?
yes
no
Muscle inflammation page 67
General condition page 82

TABLE 2.2 *Features of Arthritis Categories*

Category	*Comes on fast?*	*Typical place affected?*	*Only one part of the body?*	*Morning stiffness?*	*Fever?*
Synovitis	No	Fingers, wrists, knees	Usually many	Marked	Rare
Attachment arthritis (enthesopathy)	No	Low back, heels	Usually severe	Some	No
Crystal arthritis	Yes	Knee, ankle, big toe	Yes	No	No
Joint infection	Yes	Knee, hip, shoulder	Yes	No	Yes
Cartilage degeneration	No	End finger joints, hips, knees, neck, low back	Usually	Mild	No
Muscle inflammation	No	Muscles, not joints	No	Some	Rare
Local conditions	Yes	Elbow, shoulder, low back	Yes	No	No
General conditions	No	All over	No	No	No

arthritis or with infection of the joint. Such joints can be exquisitely painful and very warm to the touch. With synovitis, the joint inflammation is usually pretty obvious but is not quite as striking. Crystal arthritis and joint infection come on more rapidly than do the other conditions; this is what is meant by "acute." Other problems typically develop over a period of days or weeks, whereas these two problems may come on within hours.

Each of the categories typically attacks different parts of the body. Synovitis affects the knuckles, wrists, and knees. Attachment arthritis affects the low back and sometimes the heels. Crystal arthritis usually affects a knee, an ankle, or the base of the big toe. Joint infection most commonly involves a knee or other large joint. Cartilage degeneration tends to affect the joints at the end of the fingers; these joints are often spared in a synovitis. The neck can be involved by degenerative arthritis, as can the low back or the weight-bearing joints of the legs. Muscle inflammation usually spares the joints themselves. Local conditions affect only a single region. And general conditions tend to be poorly described by the patient, who often isn't sure exactly where the pain and discomfort are coming from.

All right, you know your category and can understand generally what is happening to you. Now go to the appropriate chapter and read in detail about the diseases that make up your category. The following list will help you quickly locate the section of interest.

CHAPTER 3

Synovitis
Inflammation of the Joint Membrane

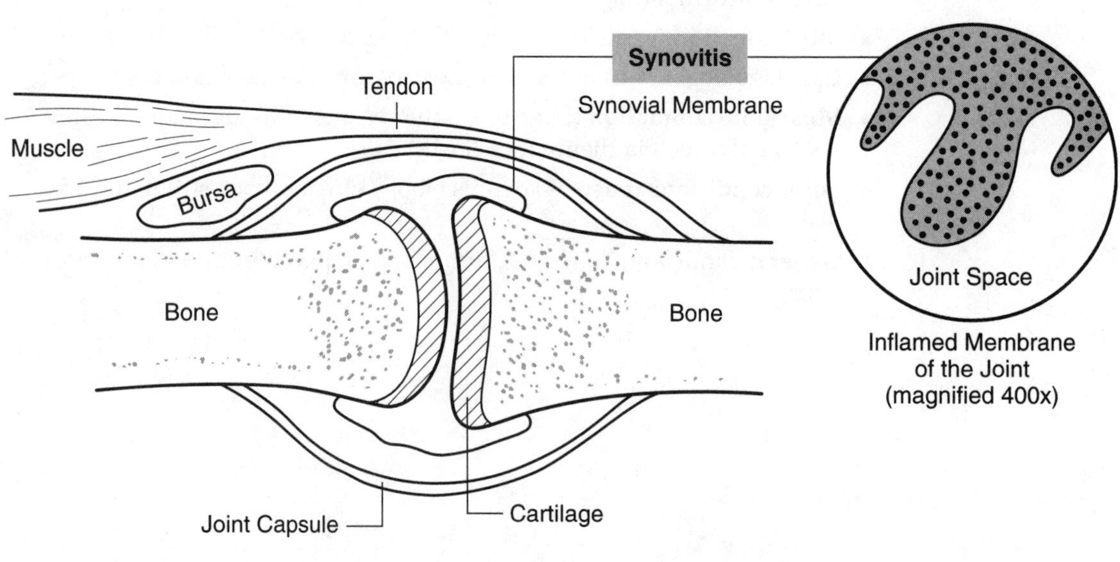

The inflammation of synovitis is located in the lining membrane of the joint, the synovium. This normally thin tissue can become more than one-quarter-inch thick due to the invasion of millions of tiny inflammatory cells. The enzymes released by the inflammation slowly digest the joint parts over many years.

Synovitis is the major problem in rheumatoid arthritis, juvenile rheumatoid arthritis, lupus, and psoriatic arthritis.

Rheumatoid Arthritis (RA)

Rheumatoid arthritis is more than just arthritis. Indeed, many doctors call it "rheumatoid disease" to emphasize the widespread nature of this process. The term *rheumatoid arthritis* is trying awkwardly to say the same thing; *rheumat* refers to the stiffness, body aching, and fatigue that are often termed "rheumatism." "Rheumatoid" means "like rheumatism." Patients with RA often describe feeling much like they have a virus, with fatigue and aching in the muscles, except that, unlike a usual viral illness, the condition may persist for months or years.

About 0.5% of our population has rheumatoid arthritis, some 1 million individuals in the United States. Most of these people (about three-quarters) are women. The condition usually appears in middle life, in the forties or fifties, although it can begin at any age. Rheumatoid arthritis in children is quite different and is described in the next section. Rheumatoid arthritis has been medically identified for about 200 years. Bone changes in the skeletons of some Mexican Indian groups suggest that the disease may have been around for thousands of years. Many, but not all, patients with RA have a particular set of genes that predispose to development of RA. Only about 1 out of 30 persons with these genes actually gets rheumatoid arthritis, so the disease seldom affects more than one family member.

Because RA is so common and can sometimes be severe, it is a major national health problem. It can result in difficulties with employment, can cause problems with daily activities, and can severely strain family relationships. In its most severe forms, and without good medical treatment, it can result in deformities of the joints and severe disability. Fortunately, many people with RA do well and lead essentially normal lives. Fear of rheumatoid arthritis, sometimes greatly exaggerated, can be as harmful as the disease itself.

Synovitis is the first and truest kind of arthritis, and rheumatoid arthritis is a perfect example of this problem. In RA the synovial membrane lining the joint becomes inflamed. We don't have a good explanation as to why this inflammation starts, but the cells in the membrane divide and grow and inflammatory cells come into the joint from other parts of the body. Because of the mass of these inflammatory cells the joint appears swollen and feels puffy or boggy to the touch. The increased blood flow that is a feature of the inflammation makes the joint warm. The cells release enzymes into the joint space and the enzymes cause further irritation and pain. Without the right medication, and if the process continues for years, these enzymes may gradually digest the cartilage and bone of the joint. Synovitis, then, is a process in which inflammation of the joint membrane, over many years, can cause damage to the joint itself.

FEATURES

Swelling and pain in one or more joints, lasting at least six weeks, is the first requirement for a diagnosis of rheumatoid arthritis. Usually both sides of the body are affected similarly and the arthritis is said to be "symmetrical." Often there are slight differences between the two sides, with the right side usually being slightly worse in right-handed people and vice versa. Occasionally the condition skips about in an erratic fashion. The wrists and knuckles are almost always involved, the knees and the joints of the ball of the foot are often involved as well, and any joint can be affected. Of the knuckles, those at the base of the fingers are most frequently painful, while the joints at the ends of the fingers are often spared. Swelling of the middle joints of the fingers often is described as "spindle-shaped" and is sometimes called *fusiform.*

Nodules, usually between the size of a pea and a mothball, may form beneath the skin in about 10% of patients. These rheumatoid nodules are most commonly located near the elbow at the place where you rest your arms on the table, but they can pop up anywhere. Each represents an inflammation of a small blood vessel. They come and go during the course of the illness and usually are not a big problem. They do tend to occur in people with the most severe kinds of RA. Rarely, they become sore or infected, particularly if they are located around the ankle. Even more rarely they form in the lungs or elsewhere in the body.

Laboratory tests sometimes can help the doctor diagnose rheumatoid arthritis. The *rheumatoid factor* or *latex* (see page 172) is the most commonly used test. Although this test may be negative in the first several months, it is eventually positive in about 80% of RA patients. The rheumatoid factor is actually an antibody to certain proteins and can sometimes be found in patients with other diseases.

The *sed rate* is another frequently used test. The full name of this test is *erythrocyte sedimentation rate,* and the name sometimes is abbreviated *ESR* (p. 170). It doesn't help in diagnosis, but it does help tell how serious the disease is. A high sed rate suggests that the disease is quite active. The joint fluid is sometimes examined in rheumatoid arthritis in order to look at the inflammatory cells or to make sure that the joint is not infected with bacteria.

X-rays (p. 176) can help the doctor determine if damage to the bones or cartilage has occurred. Some doctors like to get baseline X-rays to compare with later X-rays. It is relatively unusual for changes to be seen in the bones or cartilage in the first few months of the disease. Often it is necessary to X-ray only the hands in order to estimate the severity of the disease accurately.

Other Signs

Most patients with RA notice problems in addition to those of the joints themselves. These are usually general problems such as muscle aches, fatigue, muscle stiffness (particularly in the morning), and even a low fever. Morning stiffness is often considered a hallmark of RA and is sometimes termed the *gel phenomenon.* After a rest period or even after just sitting motionless for a few minutes, the whole body feels stiff and difficult to move. After a period of loosening up, motion becomes easier and less painful. Patients often have problems with fluid accumulation, particularly around the ankles. Occasionally the rheumatoid disease may attack other body tissues, including the whites of the eyes, the nerves, the small arteries, and the lungs. An *anemia* (low red blood cell count) is quite common, although it is seldom severe enough to require treatment.

There can be other problems due to the synovitis. A *Baker cyst* can form behind the knee and may feel like a tumor. It is just a fluid-filled joint sac, but it can extend down into the back of the calf and may cause pain like a blood clot. The *carpal tunnel syndrome* (see Wrist Pain, **S16**) involves pressure by the synovitis on a nerve at the wrist. Both of these conditions can occur in patients without rheumatoid arthritis.

Rheumatoid arthritis is one of the most complicated and mysterious diseases known. It is a challenge to patient and physician alike. Fortunately, the course of RA can be dramatically altered in most patients. More than with any other form of arthritis, you need to develop an effective partnership with your physician to combat RA's effects. A rheumatologist (joint specialist) should be involved in the treatment.

PROGNOSIS

Rheumatoid arthritis is the condition that most people think of when they hear the word arthritis. The image that comes to mind is of a person in a wheelchair, with swollen knees and twisted hands. True, most such patients have rheumatoid arthritis. Erosions of the bone itself, rupture of tendons, and slippage of the joints can be crippling. And on balance, rheumatoid arthritis is the most destructive kind of arthritis known. But most patients with rheumatoid arthritis do very much better than this. And many of the problems that do occur could have been prevented by good, early treatment.

The course of patients with RA usually falls into one of three patterns. The first, and best, is that of a brief illness lasting at most a few months and leaving no disability; this course is sometimes called *monocyclic.* The second involves a series of episodes of illness, separated by periods of being entirely well. This is sometimes termed *polycyclic* and usually does not result in very much physical impairment. The third, termed *chronic,* is a more constant disease lasting a number of years, usually for life. The great majority of patients with rheumatoid arthritis have this chronic form. Initially it is difficult to be certain which pattern will occur, but a chronic course is suggested by the presence of the rheumatoid factor on a blood test and is strongly suggested if the condition has caused problems continuously for an entire year.

Often it is hard for patients and relatives to appreciate that even the worst forms of rheumatoid arthritis can sometimes get better with time. The arthritis tends to become less aggressive. The synovitis becomes less active, and the fatigue and stiffness decrease. After several years the disease is less likely to spread to new joints. But even though the disease is less violent, any destruction of bones and ligaments that occurred in earlier years will remain. Deformities do not improve, even though no new damage is occurring. Hence, it is extremely important to treat the disease correctly in the early years, so that the joints will work well after the disease activity subsides.

TREATMENT

Treatment programs for rheumatoid arthritis are often complicated and can be confusing. In this section we broadly outline techniques for sound management. The chapters in Part II describe each treatment and provide more details. The combination of measures best for you needs to be worked out with your doctor. It has been said that the person who has himself for a doctor has a fool for a patient. In many areas of medicine, and for some kinds of arthritis, this is not true—you can do just as well looking after yourself. But with rheumatoid arthritis you do need a doctor. Indeed, with rheumatoid arthritis I strongly believe you should be seen early in the course of the disease by an arthritis specialist, a *rheumatologist*. In this way, the critical early treatment can begin at the right time. Only rheumatologists are familiar with the latest and most effective treatments.

First, some common sense. Your rheumatoid arthritis may be with you, on and off, for months or years. Think of how you want to be 20 years from now. The best treatments are those that will help you maintain a life that is as nearly normal as possible. Often the worst treatments are those that offer immediate pain relief, since they may allow joint damage to go on or may cause delayed side effects that ultimately make you feel worse. You must develop some patience with the disease and with its management. You have to adjust your thinking to operate in the same slow time frame that the disease uses. You and your doctor will want to anticipate problems before they occur so that you can avoid them. The adjustment to a long-term illness, with the necessity to plan treatment programs that may take months to get results, is a difficult psychological task. This adjustment will be one of your hardest jobs in battling your arthritis.

Synovitis is the underlying problem. Inflammation of the joint membrane releases enzymes that very slowly damage the joint structures. Good treatment reduces this inflammation and stops the damage. Painkillers can increase comfort but do not decrease the arthritis. In fact, pain actually helps to protect the joints by discouraging too much use. So in RA it is important to treat pain by treating the inflammation that causes the pain. By and large, analgesics such as codeine, Percodan, Darvon, Talwin, or Demerol must be avoided.

Rest

The proper balance between rest and exercise is an essential part of treatment. Rest reduces the inflammation, and this is good. But rest also lets joints stiffen and muscles weaken. With too much rest, tendons get weaker and bones get softer. Obviously this is bad. So moderation is the basic principle. It may help you to know that your body usually gives you the right signals about what to do and what not to do. It if hurts too much, don't do it. If you don't seem to have much problem with an activity, go ahead.

A particularly painful joint may require a splint to help it rest. Still, you will want to exercise the joint by moving it gently in different directions to prevent it from getting stiff, and you will not want to use a splint for too long—you may decide to use it only at night. As the joint gets better, begin using the joint, gently at first, but slowly progressing to more and more activity. In general, favor activities that build good muscle tone, not those that build great muscle strength. Walking and swimming are better than weight lifting, since tasks requiring a lot of strength put a lot of stress on the joint. And regular exercises done daily are better than occasional spurts of activity that stress joints not ready for so much exertion.

Common sense and a regular, long-term program are the keys to success. Should you take a nap after lunch? Yes, if you're tired. Should you undertake some particular outing? Go on a trip? You know your regular daily activity level. Common sense will answer most such questions. A return to full normal activity should be undertaken gradually, with a long-term conditioning program that includes rest when needed and graded increases in activity during nonresting periods.

Physical therapists and occupational therapists can often help with specific advice and helpful hints. The best therapists will help you develop your own program for home exercise and will teach you the exercises and activities that will help your joints. However, don't expect the therapist to do your program for you. Your rest and exercise program cannot consist solely of formal sessions at a rehabilitation facility. You must take the responsibility to build the habits that will, on a daily basis, protect and strengthen your joints. We have provided many of these hints and suggestions in this book's companion volume, *The Arthritis Helpbook,* and you may wish to obtain a copy.

Medications

Medications are required by almost all patients with rheumatoid arthritis, and often must be continued for years. Great progress has been made recently with disease-modifying antirheumatic drugs (DMARDs), bringing about a virtual revolution in the treatment of rheumatoid arthritis (see page 140). These crucial drugs should be prescribed early in the course of the disease. The most important rule now is: "Don't do too little, too late." The traditional DMARDs are Plaquenil, Azulfidine, gold shots, oral gold, penicillamine, methotrexate, Imuran, and cyclosporine. The new DMARDs are leflunomide and the anti–tumor necrosis factor drugs, and these are substantial advances. They are discussed in Chapter 15. The great majority of patients with RA should be taking one or a combination of DMARDs at all times.

Antimalarial drugs such as chloroquine or Plaquenil (p. 146) are often used as the first DMARDs. Gold injections (p. 142) are often very helpful and sometimes result in complete disappearance of the arthritis if used early enough. Penicillamine (p. 145) can also bring dramatic improvement. Auranofin (Ridaura, p. 144) and sulphasalazine (Azulfidine, p. 147) are more recent additions to this drug category, and both are major advances.

Aspirin and the nonsteroidal anti-inflammatory drugs (NSAIDs) are described in detail in Chapter 14. They can be useful, but remember that the DMARDs are the most important medications. Every patient with RA should become familiar with the uses of aspirin, which, used correctly (p. 115), is a good analgesic drug with an acceptable level of side effects. Aspirin variants, such as Disalcid and Trilisate, may better protect the stomach lining. The new drugs Celebrex, Vioxx, Mobic, and nabumetone have better safety records than most of the older drugs.

Corticosteroids, most frequently prednisone (p. 137), are strong hormones with formidable long-term side effects. Their use is controversial in rheumatoid arthritis; some physicians feel they should almost never be used; others use them only in very small doses.

Immunosuppressant drugs such as Imuran (p. 151) and methotrexate (p. 150) are powerful. Methotrexate is now recognized to be the most effective of these strong drugs and is quite well tolerated. Imuran also is well tolerated by most people, but it is not always as effective. The anti-TNF drugs Remicade and Enbrel are expensive and difficult to use but are very powerful. Leflunomide now provides an alternative to methotrexate.

Surgery sometimes can restore the function of a damaged joint. Hip replacement, knee replacement, shoulder replacement, synovectomy of the knee, metatarsal head resection, and synovectomy of the knuckles are among the most frequent operations; these are discussed in Chapter 17.

If you have rheumatoid arthritis, proceed to Part II, page 103.

Arthritis in Children (Juvenile Rheumatoid Arthritis, JRA)

Children get arthritis too. In fact, over 30,000 children in the United States have an important kind of arthritis called *juvenile rheumatoid arthritis (JRA).* This name, however, is misleading, since it suggests that these children have a disease similar to rheumatoid arthritis in adults. For the most part these children have a quite different set of problems and require quite different treatment. The outlook for their complete recovery is much better than that of persons with adult rheumatoid arthritis.

Children, of course, lead very active lives and continually put stresses on their joints, muscles, and back. They fall down, sprain their ankles, and experience a variety of temporary aches and pains that are not really arthritis. Occasionally a child will be born with an abnormality in a knee, hip, or elsewhere. Again, this is not really arthritis. Very rarely, a child will have a joint infected with bacteria (most commonly the *Staphylococcus*), which causes a severe infectious arthritis like that discussed later (p. 52). An adolescent will sometimes develop arthritis due to infection with gonococcal bacteria. These problems are true arthritis, but they are acute forms. They develop rapidly and last less than six weeks. In this section we are concerned with arthritis of longer duration in children.

Three forms of juvenile arthritis are now generally recognized. The first, *monoarticular arthritis,* occurs in only one joint or, at most, in two, three, or four joints. The second, *systemic arthritis,* is more impressive for its high fever and its skin rash than for the arthritis itself. The third, *polyarticular arthritis,* involves many joints and resembles the rheumatoid arthritis seen in adults.

Beyond these major subtypes, there are other kinds of chronic arthritis in children. Acute rheumatic fever is a completely different disease that must not be confused with other forms of childhood arthritis. And some kinds of attachment arthritis described in Chapter 4, such as ankylosing spondylitis, can occur in adolescents.

FEATURES

The following paragraphs describe the features of the three types of juvenile arthritis, and acute rheumatic fever.

Monoarticular juvenile arthritis simply means juvenile arthritis that involves only one joint. Most frequently this joint is a knee. *Pauciarticular* and *oligoarticular* are similar words that mean "few joints" and allow for the fact that this type of arthritis may involve one, two, three, or even four joints. Usually the joints involved are large ones. Most children with pauciarticular arthritis feel generally well except for their swollen, sore, affected joints. In a few instances there may be involvement of the eye.

Many doctors will ask an ophthalmologist to perform periodically a *slit lamp* examination of the eye to detect any eye problems. In this procedure, a thin beam of light is projected obliquely onto the eye through a narrow slit to permit examination of the eye by a magnifying lens.

The *systemic* form of juvenile arthritis is far more dramatic. This form has been called *Still's disease.* A child may suddenly develop a very high fever, as high as 106°F (41°C), and may be very ill with fatigue, muscle aching, and perhaps a fine, red skin rash. The liver, spleen, and lymph nodes may be enlarged, and the disease may involve other organs as well. The attack may last days or weeks and disappear as quickly and mysteriously as it came. A few months or years later it may recur again and again and again. With the initial attack there may be just a little arthritis, quite a bit of arthritis, or no arthritis at all. Eventually arthritis will accompany every attack, but this may not occur for several years.

Polyarticular juvenile arthritis affects many joints and usually comes on slowly in children approaching adolescence. The arthritis is usually experienced equally on both sides of the body and frequently affects the wrists and knuckles as well as the knees and other joints. This form is characterized by intense inflammation of the joint membrane (synovitis), and closely resembles the rheumatoid arthritis seen in adults.

Acute rheumatic fever follows a streptococcal infection, usually a "strep throat." It is a much less frequent illness now than it was a few years ago. The possibility of acute rheumatic fever is the major reason that throat cultures are taken and that penicillin is sometimes given to treat sore throats, since rheumatic fever can be prevented by such treatment. Acute rheumatic fever is an allergic (immunologic) reaction of the body against a strep bacteria infection that occurred several weeks earlier. Antibodies attack the joints, and sometimes the heart valves and other parts of the body.

The arthritis of rheumatic fever is termed *migratory.* It will, for example, appear in one joint, such as the knee, then migrate to a shoulder, then to a wrist, and then to the other knee. Affected children may have a heart murmur, a fever, or an unusual red skin rash with sharp, irregular borders.

Tests

Laboratory tests for juvenile arthritis are not very helpful. By and large, all of the usual tests for arthritis are negative. Even in children with the polyarticular arthritis most closely resembling adult rheumatoid arthritis, only a minority have a positive rheumatoid-factor test. The sedimentation rate (p. 170) is often elevated, but this indicates the severity of the inflammation and not the accuracy of the diagnosis. With acute rheumatic fever, a blood test can confirm that a streptococcal infection has occurred recently.

Similarly, X-rays are usually not very helpful. This is a fortunate thing, since we do not like to X-ray children unnecessarily. Destruction of the joints sufficient to cause X-ray changes to the bone is uncommon in children. Watching the course of the disease with time often provides the most important diagnostic clues. Does the arthritis stay in the original joints? Are there associated skin rashes or fever? Does the arthritis come in recurring attacks? Does it tend to involve both sides of the body equally? Such questions, repeated over time, require patience on the part of parent, child, and physician. The patience is usually rewarded by a good outcome for the child.

PROGNOSIS

Many of us have the idea that arthritis, once encountered, is present for life. This is not true. When a child develops arthritis, the concern of parents, child, and even the child's school is naturally intense. Fortunately, in children the disease usually disappears entirely with time. Most children with juvenile arthritis will grow into normal adults without any leftover bone or joint problems. This does not mean that parent or child can relax. Hard work is required to prevent development of permanent stiffness, particularly when a period of active arthritis coincides with one of rapid growth. The long-term outlook, however, is good.

This is particularly true of the first two categories of juvenile arthritis. At least two-thirds of children with monoarticular or pauciarticular disease will have no problems with arthritis as adults. Even with the dramatic systemic form (Still's disease) a similar two-thirds of children will have no problems as adults. The outlook is not quite as favorable for children with polyarticular arthritis; about half of these children will continue to require treatment for arthritis in adult life.

Acute rheumatic fever does not cause joint destruction, and arthritis continuing into adult life is unusual.

TREATMENT

Medications

Drug treatment of arthritis in children centers around the use of NSAIDs (p. 112). Aspirin, an anti-inflammatory, in appropriate doses, will satisfactorily control the arthritis in the great majority of patients. Some of the new anti-inflammatory agents are also useful and may be safer, but not all are yet approved for use in children. Tylenol is safe and is frequently used; aspirin should be avoided in children with fever.

On the other hand, the bad effects of the corticosteroids (p. 135) on childhood growth are well understood; these agents stop bone growth and can lead to failure to reach adult height. Other side effects of steroids also occur; thus, these drugs must be used with extreme caution in growing children. Their most justifiable use is in short courses of treatment for the dramatic but brief episodes of illness with Still's disease, or occasionally for severe eye problems.

The careful physician relies on aspirin or other nonsteroidal anti-inflammatory drugs (NSAIDs) as the major medication for pauciarticular disease. Parents, child, and physician must always take the long view. An exception is that with very high fever, chicken pox, or influenza, most doctors now avoid or discontinue aspirin because of the possibility of triggering a severe liver and neurologic condition known as Reye syndrome.

Methotrexate is now being used more frequently in children with polyarticular disease, as are the other DMARDs.

Exercise

Physical therapy and exercise programs, particularly swimming, are very helpful in maintaining muscle tone and mobility in the child with arthritis. Sometimes special arrangements with the child's school are required so that the child doesn't fall behind during the time the arthritis is expected to remain active. Since the overall outlook is good a reasonable plan of management includes attention to keeping the child up with his or her peers, so that when the arthritis subsides a normal school and social pattern can be resumed. For many patients, body contact sports and activities (such as basketball) that require a lot of jumping should be discouraged, but only while the disease is active.

Surgery

Surgery is seldom required, and indications for surgery are similar to those in adults. It is needed only infrequently because the destructive aspects of the arthritis are less severe in children. Surgical removal of the synovium (joint membrane) of the knee is sometimes required, but this is performed less frequently now than a few years ago. "Soft tissue release" procedures to increase motion (capsulotomy) are fairly frequently performed.

Rather rarely, removal of joint fluid through a needle provides some relief. Sometimes injection of a corticosteroid preparation into a knee joint or other joint is helpful. Since too many treatments of this kind can accelerate bone destruction, they must be used with caution.

If childhood arthritis is the problem, proceed to Part II, page 103.

Lupus (Systemic Lupus Erythematosus, SLE)

The word *lupus* means "wolf." The disease is so named because some lupus patients develop a red rash across the nose and cheeks that causes the face to look a little bit like that of a wolf. The full name of the disease, *systemic lupus erythematosus,* is a bit hard to remember. *Systemic* refers to the many parts of the body that may be involved by this condition. *Erythema* refers to the red color of the rash. There is a skin condition with a somewhat similar rash called *discoid lupus erythematosus;* thus, the word *systemic* serves to emphasize that SLE is a more widespread disease.

Lupus is not always thought of as a form of arthritis. Lupus is described as a "connective-tissue" disease or a "collagen" disease or a "collagen vascular" disease. These terms describe a family of diseases discussed further starting on page 89. About half of lupus patients have arthritis.

Lupus is also considered an *autoimmune* disease—that is, most of the problems seem to come from antibodies created by the body attacking other parts of the body. In the case of the arthritis, the body is using its defense systems intended for outside viruses to attack the lining of its own joints.

This is a highly variable disease. Some patients with lupus aren't even aware they have it and require no treatment. Others have a major illness. Lupus has developed a much worse reputation than it deserves, since newspaper, magazine, and television depictions of the disease focus on those relatively few patients with dramatic symptoms rather than on the many who do well without major difficulties.

FEATURES

The arthritis of lupus is a synovitis; it involves inflammation of the membrane lining the joint. Compared with rheumatoid arthritis, however, the synovitis is less severe. Whereas the patient with rheumatoid arthritis usually has visibly swollen joints that feel spongy to the touch, the joints of a patient with lupus arthritis may appear entirely normal. When we look at the synovial membrane under the microscope, we see that the thick *pannus* (covering membrane) of inflammatory tissue so characteristic of rheumatoid arthritis is not present. Rather, there is a less violent inflammation of the joint membrane. This difference in intensity of the inflammatory response is one reason why the arthritis of lupus is usually not as severe as rheumatoid arthritis.

The joints affected by lupus are almost exactly the same ones affected by rheumatoid arthritis. The wrists, the knuckles at the base of the fingers, the knuckles in the middle of the fingers, and the knees are most commonly involved. Sometimes the hips may be attacked, and on occasion there is a problem with the blood supply to the hip or other joints, causing a complication called *aseptic necrosis.* Although these are the joints most often affected, any joint in the body may be involved. The spine is usually spared.

The usual symptom is pain. The joints will be tender when squeezed and sore when moved. As noted, they may not look abnormal at all. The doctor may initially be skeptical about the presence of arthritis, but laboratory tests will help confirm the existence of the disease.

X-rays of the arthritis of lupus are usually normal. In rheumatoid arthritis the inflammatory process actually erodes the bones causing little holes to develop near the ends of the bones. With lupus these erosions are very rare, and it is unusual for the arthritis to damage the joint very much.

Other Signs

We are currently following about four hundred patients with lupus, and each has had evidence of abnormal antibodies. Additionally, each has had disease of at least two body systems out of the six listed below. Most of these problems are mild or last only a short period.

The *skin* may be affected with rashes or sores. Sometimes there is Raynaud's phenomenon, in which the fingers become blue and white after exposure to cold. Small ulcers may develop inside the mouth. The skin rash may take a characteristic butterfly appearance over the cheeks, and it may become worse after exposure to sunlight.

The *blood* elements may be affected by the antibodies of lupus. The white cells are frequently decreased, a condition termed *leukopenia.* The red cells may be depressed (*anemia*) by an antibody reaction or just by the general effects of the disease. The platelets may be severely depressed (*thrombocytopenia*), leading to bleeding.

The *pleura* that surrounds the lungs, the *pericardium* that surrounds the heart, and the *peritoneum* that surrounds the abdominal cavity are called *serous membranes.* Each of these may be inflamed at times in lupus, the pleura being the most commonly affected (*pleurisy*).

The *lungs* may, rather rarely, be involved in lupus. This problem resembles a mild pneumonia, but it is not caused by germs and clears with anti-inflammatory drugs and without antibiotics.

The *kidneys* pose a major problem with lupus, and at least half of patients with lupus have some kidney difficulty. Lupus causes *nephritis* when the antibodies form *immune complexes* that collect inside the kidneys.

The *central nervous system* is involved every so often in lupus. Seizures or other nervous or emotional problems may result.

Tests

Because lupus is an immunological disease, the diagnosis can be assisted by the finding of antibodies in the blood. The most common blood test detects *antinuclear antibodies,* which are found in some other diseases but are most characteristic of lupus. This blood test is positive in almost everyone with lupus. Sometimes the sedimentation rate will be elevated, there may be a low white blood count, and many other blood tests may be abnormal.

PROGNOSIS

The arthritis of lupus has a good prognosis. Doctors usually talk about it as being "nondeforming," meaning that injury to the bone is rare and that patients usually do well over a long period without any crippling. On the other hand, the arthritis does tend to be persistent and may remain active for many months or years. Ultimately, the activity of the disease begins to subside, but this may require five, ten, or even fifteen years.

A few patients with lupus arthritis do develop some deformity of the joints, particularly of the hands. These deformities are somewhat different from those of rheumatoid arthritis because they result from slippage, or *subluxation,* of the joints rather than destruction of the bone ends. The tendons and ligaments around the joint get a little loose, and a certain degree of deformity may result. For example, the fingers may bend backward more than they should, or a finger may be bent backward at the middle knuckle and forward at the last knuckle, giving the appearance of a "swan neck." Usually the hand will work well even if this problem occurs; serious disability resulting from the arthritis is unusual.

Only a small fraction of all of the things that can possibly happen in lupus will happen to any one person. Patients frequently worry unrealistically about what might go wrong next. The prognosis in lupus has improved now, so that death from the disease is quite unusual. More than 90% of all patients with lupus live at least ten years after the onset of the disease, and the majority live normal life spans. The prognosis depends on the particular kind of lupus. Patients who have the arthritis of lupus or who have the Raynaud's phenomenon (color changes in the hands after exposure to cold) do somewhat better than the average lupus patient, while those who have involvement of the kidneys or central nervous system do a bit worse. But the outlook is now much better for all.

TREATMENT

Treatment of lupus is complicated, since the disease varies considerably from one person to another. Powerful and dangerous drugs such as corticosteroids (p. 135) and immunosuppressants (p. 149) in high doses are required for some patients with SLE. However, the disease can usually be managed with either low doses of corticosteroids, aspirin (p. 115) or other anti-inflammatory agents, hydroxychloroquine (p. 146), or other reasonably safe drugs. Perhaps a quarter of lupus patients require little treatment and may do better without even these mild drugs.

Lifestyle, as in all of the rheumatic diseases, can make a significant difference in the effectiveness of a treatment program. Worry can become as serious a malady as the disease itself. While certainty about prognosis is not always possible, the odds are good for every patient and minimum disruption in lifestyle is the goal.

The tendency in past years to counsel strict avoidance of the sun and strict avoidance of overactivity has now been greatly relaxed. We urge patients to stay out of the sun only if being out in the sun causes a flare-up of their disease, and to rest only if they are tired. We have been rewarded with many patients living confident, productive lives who, in more restrictive years, would have been socially quarantined.

Knowledge that the arthritis is unlikely to result in crippling and that the great majority of patients can lead essentially normal lives is very helpful to many patients. A good long-term relationship with a physician familiar with this disease is important. The physician will want to follow the patient to ensure that complicating disease of other body organs does not occur.

Surgery is seldom required. Occasionally operations to realign the tendons of the finger joints are performed. And if aseptic necrosis of the hip has developed, surgery of the hip joint—usually total replacement of the hip—is sometimes required.

If you have lupus, proceed to Part II, page 103.

Psoriatic Arthritis

The skin condition psoriasis is well known to most people because it is so common. Red scaling patches, which sometimes bleed when injured, are common near the elbows and knees but can occur anyplace on the body. Often the fingernails or an area around the fingernails is affected with these psoriatic skin patches. In cases of extensive psoriasis, much of the body may be covered with the skin lesions. In psoriasis, the lower layers of the skin contain cells that divide more rapidly than normal, causing patches of thicker skin to grow and then scale off from the top.

It is not as well known that arthritis can occur with psoriasis. Probably some 10% of patients with psoriasis also have some arthritis. Arthritis experts have argued for years about the exact forms of arthritis that can accompany psoriasis, and the picture is not yet totally clear. Nevertheless, there is agreement that particular types of arthritis are directly related to the skin condition.

Part of the confusion is caused by the fact that both psoriasis and several forms of arthritis are quite common. Hence, just as a matter of coincidence, you would expect to see some people with both psoriasis and arthritis. This will, of course, be most common with the most frequently occurring forms of arthritis: ankylosing spondylitis, rheumatoid arthritis, gout, and osteoarthritis. If your arthritis closely resembles one of these types, it may not be psoriatic arthritis at all, even though you may have both psoriasis and arthritis.

FEATURES

Psoriatic arthritis is part synovitis and part attachment arthritis, so it is discussed here, immediately preceding the next chapter on attachment arthritis.

In contrast with rheumatoid arthritis, psoriatic arthritis is usually not the same on both sides of the body, and it affects different sets of joints. Whereas rheumatoid arthritis affects the middle knuckles more frequently, psoriatic arthritis often attacks the end joints of the fingers. The joints involved by psoriatic arthritis are frequently spotty and irregular in their distribution. For example, the second finger of one hand and the third finger and thumb of the other hand might be affected.

Rheumatoid arthritis frequently results in overall tiredness and fatigue, with pronounced stiffness in the morning and with wasting of the calcium in the bones. In psoriatic arthritis these features are less common. The patient frequently feels perfectly well except for the problems with the skin and joints, and is not excessively fatigued. Further, bone strength usually is preserved throughout the course of the disease.

Some patients with psoriatic arthritis will experience an unusual feature of the disease termed a "sausage digit." This is a finger or a toe swollen uniformly from beginning to end, so that it resembles a sausage. It may be twice the size of an adjacent finger or toe. This results from synovitis of the joints of the digit together with swelling of the soft tissues between the joints. The sausage digit occurs only in psoriatic arthritis and in the condition called Reiter's syndrome, discussed in Chapter 4.

Pain in the heel or low back pain sometimes accompanies psoriatic arthritis, although these problems are unusual in rheumatoid arthritis. In some patients the joint problems will come and go as the skin problem worsens or improves; this relationship is not constant.

Tests

There are no good laboratory tests for psoriatic arthritis. The skin disease is usually easily identified on sight by physical examination, but it can be confirmed by looking at a biopsy of skin under the microscope. Blood tests for the rheumatoid factor (*latex fixation*) are usually negative. The sedimentation rate may be elevated or not.

X-rays may show bone erosions similar to those of rheumatoid arthritis. More characteristic, however, is the formation of new bone along the sides of existing bones, giving a fluffy X-ray appearance. Erosions sometimes result in "whittling" of the ends of the bones so that a bone end that should be approximately square develops a point almost like a pencil. X-rays of the back may show changes similar to ankylosing spondylitis in the sacroiliac joints and in the spine. However, involvement of the sacroiliac joints is often spotty; only one side may be involved or the two sides may be involved but with different degrees of severity. When involvement of the spine occurs, just one side of a particular vertebra may be affected.

PROGNOSIS

Throughout this book there is an emphasis on the variability in prognosis for arthritis. It is important to realize that very few patients are severely crippled by arthritis. Psoriatic arthritis easily wins the distinction of being the most variable of all of the rheumatic diseases. In the great majority of patients the disease is mild; it might even be termed trivial. Medication may be required at some times and there may be some stiffness in one or another joint, but the arthritis is not as severe a problem as the skin.

On the other hand, in the very worst cases a condition that is probably the most crippling arthritis of all occurs. This condition is called *arthritis mutilans.* It is a very rare happening, affecting less than 0.1% of all patients with psoriasis and arthritis, and should not pose a major worry for most patients. Some *arthritis mutilans* patients have a combination of the worst possibilities of rheumatoid arthritis and ankylosing spondylitis. We believe that the worst outcomes usually can now be prevented by correct early treatment.

Because fatigue, tiredness, and stiffness are less prominent in psoriatic arthritis than in rheumatoid arthritis, almost all patients are able to work and play normally throughout their lives. Relatively few will have difficulty with employment, with homemaking, or with most of their other daily activities.

TREATMENT

Patients should maintain a schedule of essentially normal activities unless a particular problem mandates some limitation. Techniques of protecting involved joints are important, as is exercising these joints through their entire range of motion to prevent stiffening. Resting the entire body, sometimes important in rheumatoid arthritis, is seldom needed, and fatigue is usually not present. Beyond this, the same general treatment principles apply as for rheumatoid arthritis.

Drug treatment for psoriatic arthritis has a slightly different spectrum from that of rheumatoid arthritis. Indomethacin (p. 124), Naprosyn (p. 128), and other anti-inflammatory agents frequently are better than aspirin for this condition. Corticosteroids (p. 135) such as prednisone are not frequently useful in psoriatic arthritis. Although the skin condition may improve temporarily with these drugs, it sometimes becomes worse on discontinuation of the steroid. Most doctors try to avoid these drugs whenever possible. Controversy reigns concerning the use of gold shots (p. 142). Some physicians are of the opinion that gold injections may increase the skin disease while others use these injections frequently and apparently safely.

For severe cases, the immunosuppressant drugs, particularly methotrexate (p. 150) and azathioprine (p. 151), are often used. In psoriatic arthritis they have the advantage of being effective against both the skin and the joint problems. Since psoriatic arthritis patients are constitutionally strong, these powerful drugs are usually well tolerated with few side effects.

Finally, one may treat psoriatic arthritis by treating the psoriasis. Since in some patients there is a linkage between the state of the skin disease and the state of the arthritis, aggressive treatment efforts using appropriate tars, creams, drugs, and ultraviolet light are sometimes successful in reducing the level of activity of the arthritis.

If your problem is psoriatic arthritis, proceed to Part II, page 103.

CHAPTER 4

Attachment Arthritis

Inflammation of the Joint Attachments

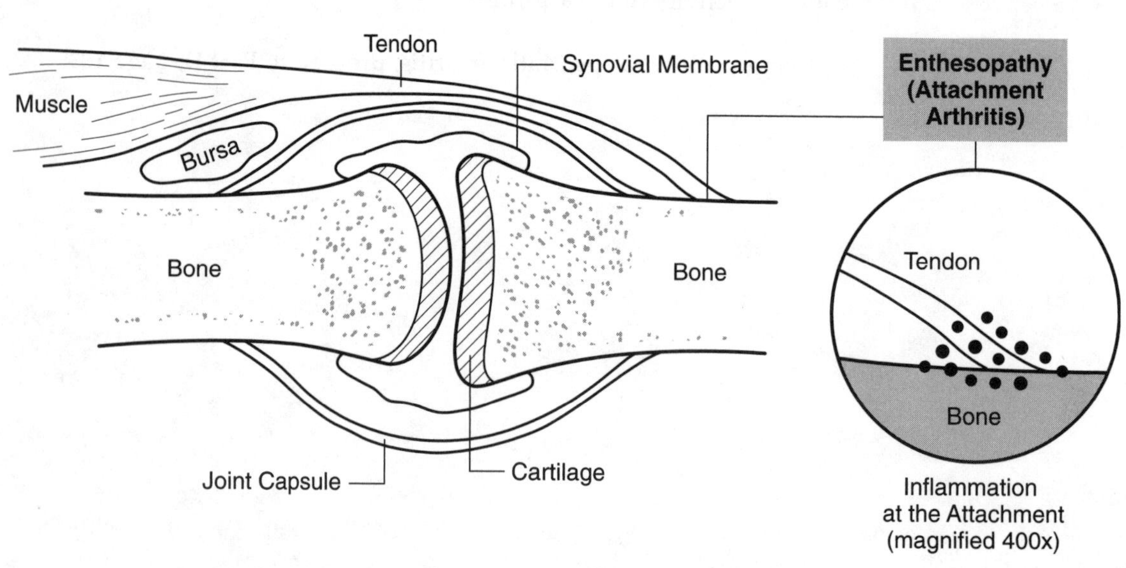

Inflammation at the Attachment (magnified 400x)

The inflammation of an **enthesopathy** is located where a ligament or a tendon attaches to the bone. The small dark inflammatory cells invade this area and cause pain and tissue damage. For this book, we introduce the term **attachment arthritis** in place of the more technical term **enthesopathy** to explain this process.

Ankylosing spondylitis, Reiter's syndrome, and sometimes psoriatic arthritis or arthritis associated with bowel disease are forms of attachment arthritis. These diseases are related to a particular gene and run in families.

Ankylosing Spondylitis (AS)

Ankylosing spondylitis has a jawbreaker of a name. This disease has gone by a variety of other names during the 3,000 years that it is known to have existed as a human disease. In this century, it was first called Marie-Strumpel disease, after the two doctors who first described the condition fully. Later it became known as rheumatoid spondylitis. Since this name suggested that it was related to rheumatoid arthritis, which it is not, the name has been changed to ankylosing spondylitis, or AS for short. Most recently it has been called simply spondylitis.

A "poker spine" is the feature of this disease that most people are familiar with. Severely affected patients have a very stiff back, like a poker, and are unable to bend. Unlike rheumatoid arthritis, which affects the joints of the hands and feet, ankylosing spondylitis affects the central parts of the body. More importantly, the disease is distinguished from rheumatoid arthritis by being an *enthesopathy,* or attachment arthritis, instead of a synovitis. I use the term *attachment arthritis* in place of *enthesopathy* simply because it is easier to understand. Your doctor will be familiar with the condition but possibly not with the new term.

The inflammation in attachment arthritis is not in the lining membrane of the joint but rather where the ligaments and tendons attach to the bone, right next to the joint. Understanding this difference will make clear why spondylitis affects certain parts of the body, why it causes stiffness more than pain, and why it responds to different medicines from those used for rheumatoid arthritis.

Ankylosing spondylitis is a genetic disease. The gene region that predisposes to ankylosing spondylitis has been identified; it is on the sixth chromosome. This disease tends to occur in families; over one-half of patients with ankylosing spondylitis have another family member with the disease. The gene region associated with the disease is called *B27.* If you have the gene, our data suggest that you may have as high as a 20% chance of developing ankylosing spondylitis or a related "reactive arthritis" at some time during your life. If you don't have the gene, for all practical purposes you are immune to ankylosing spondylitis. Nearly 100% of white patients with ankylosing spondylitis have this gene; the proportion is lower in blacks.

About 7% of white individuals in the United States carry the B27 gene region. Thus, ankylosing spondylitis is a common disease that may occur in as much as 1% of the population of the United States. Genetic factors are often closely associated with race, and B27 is no exception. Some North American Indian tribes have as much as 50% frequency of the gene, and these Indian tribes have a very high frequency of spondylitis. B27 is very rare among blacks, and the disease almost never affects black individuals.

Identification of the gene region is allowing research on this disease to proceed at a rapid pace. It seems likely that the cause of this form of arthritis will be known within a few years, permitting even more effective treatment. It is likely that the condition is a reaction by the immune system of susceptible individuals to a bacterium that lives in the large bowel of many people. B27-positive individuals tend to develop a reactive arthritis after exposure to certain bacteria, including *Shigella, Salmonella, Yersinia, Chlamydia,* and perhaps *Klebsiella.*

FEATURES

Not all of the joints of the body have a synovial lining. Some consist simply of fibers that bridge across the joint and allow limited movement. Since ankylosing spondylitis is an attachment arthritis, it affects such joints more than those with the synovial lining. The sacroiliac (SI) joint attaches the sacrum at the bottom of the spine to the pelvic bones by means of many strong fibers. Thus, it is not surprising that the sacroiliac joints are those most involved in ankylosing spondylitis. Sacroiliitis is the hallmark of this disease, and almost all patients have sacroiliac-caused back pain. The pain usually has a component of stiffness, and the stiffness is worse in the morning. The disease comes on slowly, usually beginning around age 20. The back pain usually is not associated with any accident or injury.

Over time the condition tends to move from the lower regions of the spine toward the higher. It may involve the fibrous joints that attach the ribs to the spine and the ribs to the breastbone. It may reach the neck. If it extends to the joints of the limbs, usually just the hips or perhaps the shoulders are involved. In severe cases, the attachment of the skull to the neck can be ankylosed and frozen.

The inflammation at the ends of the ligaments results in stiffness and pain with movement. After a period of stiffness and pain, a bony bridge grows between the bones that make up the joint and the area becomes totally rigid. Obviously this fusion stops motion, but it has the beneficial effect of removing pain; pain is experienced only in areas that are still able to move. Rheumatoid arthritis can cause destruction of the bones around a joint, whereas ankylosing spondylitis fuses the intact bones together.

Tests

The most important diagnostic test of AS is an X-ray of the sacroiliac joints (p. 177). Usually the disease, if it has been present for two years or longer, can be conclusively diagnosed by a single X-ray of the pelvis with particular attention paid to the state of the sacroiliac joints.

When the doctor is examining the patient, stiffness in the back may be measured by tests of back flexion. The chest may not expand as fully as it should because of involvement of the joints at the ends of the ribs. This can be detected by putting a tape measure around the chest at the level of the nipples and noting the difference between the chest circumference after the biggest possible intake of breath and after blowing all of the air out of the chest. Normally the chest circumference changes by at least two inches (5 cm), but many patients with ankylosing spondylitis will have a change of less than one-half inch (1 cm). Such simple tests can strongly suggest a diagnosis of AS, but X-rays are required to confirm it.

In contrast, other tests are not as helpful. Almost all laboratory tests are normal. The sedimentation rate is elevated in some patients but is normal in others. The B27 test for the underlying gene (p. 173) will be positive in almost everyone. The problem with this test is that, since the gene is found in 7% of the white population, a positive test for the gene does not necessarily prove ankylosing spondylitis. Most people with the B27 gene are well.

Other Signs

In a few patients, particularly those who are most severely affected, ankylosing spondylitis can cause an inflammation of the eye with redness and pain, may result in damage to the aortic valve of the heart, or may be associated with cavities in the lungs. In severely affected patients, when the rib cage does not move well, pneumonia may develop.

The bony fusion can be extensive in the most severely affected patients and can lead to the creation of a single giant bone that includes the pelvis, the spine, the skull, and the ribs, without any motion at all in the central part of the body. The fusion is usually symmetrical, with both sacroiliac joints involved to the same extent and with both sides of the spine and rib cage equally involved.

PROGNOSIS

Ankylosing spondylitis is most frequently a mild condition and is not considered a serious problem by either patient or physician. For example, the diagnosis is often not made until around age 40, while the disease began some 20 years earlier. Some studies suggest that there are ten times as many patients with ankylosing spondylitis who are undiagnosed in the United States as there are patients who have been diagnosed. Early studies that suggested the disease is found almost entirely in men have come under some attack; it is now felt that the disease may be nearly as common in women, although in a milder form.

Almost all patients with ankylosing spondylitis lead vigorous, physically active lives without major limitation from the disease. Patients with spondylitis usually have better than normal employment records without undue absences. Even complete fusion of the back is consistent with a nearly normal lifestyle. Patients with ankylosing spondylitis usually adapt very well to the presence of a chronic disease and do not experience major difficulties.

Probably fewer than one out of one hundred patients with spondylitis progress to serious limitation or deformity. Death due to the disease is very unusual and almost all patients have a normal life span. Death can occasionally occur from a severe problem with the aortic valve or from a serious infection of the lungs, but only in those few patients who have the most severe forms of the disease.

The most common significant limitation is a fusion of the neck in a flexed position, limiting the person's ability to raise the head. The hips are involved in a small percentage of patients, and if this involvement is serious, limitation of mobility may result.

TREATMENT

The approach to treatment follows logically from the discussion above. Since the disease is working to fuse parts of the body together, the therapeutic response involves stretching those body parts. Motion exercises with stretching in all directions should be performed several times daily. Many physicians recommend deep-breathing exercises in order to slow the fusion of the rib joints. Posture is as important as exercise. Patients should sleep on their back without a pillow so that the spine is rested in the most useful position; even if fusion occurs, it will happen in the position of best function. Using good chairs and other commonsense measures are important. I have seen patients who could sleep only on one side and who used several pillows develop a neck deformity with the head cocked to one side. Clearly this could have been avoided.

Anticipating the possibility that the motion of the chest might be limited at some point, we urge patients to stop cigarette smoking, since smoking can damage the lungs and aggravate the later tendency to develop lung infections.

Since this is a genetic disease, many patients ask about the risk to other family members or about the advisability of having children. While these decisions must be made by the individual, medical advice is reassuring. If an individual with ankylosing spondylitis is married to an individual who is negative for the B27 gene, then any particular child has a one in two chance of carrying the gene and a one in ten chance of developing the disease. Of family members who may be affected, most will have mild and almost undetectable disease. Since the gene appears to cause no other form of illness and since patients with ankylosing spondylitis are frequently noteworthy for their good general health, there seems little reason to counsel patients not to have a family.

The symptoms of ankylosing spondylitis can be strikingly decreased by medical treatment, and patients with ankylosing spondylitis should be under medical treatment as long as they are experiencing pain or stiffness. Indomethacin (p. 124) and naproxen (p. 128) are among the more useful drugs. Aspirin (p. 115) does not seem to be as helpful in ankylosing spondylitis as it is in rheumatoid arthritis, and it is used less frequently. Corticosteroids should be used very seldom for this disease. Methotrexate and other DMARDs are now used more commonly in severely affected patients.

There is medical controversy as to whether these drugs actually prevent the fusion of bones. The drugs do relieve symptoms in most patients at any stage of the disease. Over the short term—weeks or months—they clearly improve the motion of the spine and allow the patient to exercise to a wider range of motion. No adequate studies of the long-term effects of these drugs have been performed, but reports suggest that patients who have had regular medical treatment end up with much less stiffness than those who have not. The control of symptoms allows greater degrees of motion.

For people with severe hip involvement, total hip replacement surgery is sometimes required and can be very helpful.

If you have ankylosing spondylitis, proceed to Part II, page 103.

Reiter's Syndrome

A German army physician, Hans Reiter, first described this syndrome during World War I. Reiter described a disease with three features—an arthritis, a painful inflammation of the eye (*conjunctivitis*), and a discharge from the penis (*urethritis*)—in an army lieutenant. Later observers added a fourth feature sometimes characteristic of the disease, a particular skin rash called *keratoderma blennorrhagica.* Reiter's syndrome is relatively rare compared to most of the forms of arthritis described in this book, but it is the second most common cause of arthritis in young men in their late teens or twenties. (Ankylosing spondylitis is the first.) Reiter's syndrome is almost always a disease of men.

The same gene (B27) that is almost always present in ankylosing spondylitis is usually present in Reiter's syndrome. Reiter's patients have this gene from 70% to 90% of the time, compared with 7% in the general white population. (Like ankylosing spondylitis, Reiter's syndrome is unusual among blacks.) Occasionally members of the same family may have the disease, underscoring the genetic effect, but family members are more likely to have ankylosing spondylitis than the rarer Reiter's syndrome.

Infections seem to cause Reiter's syndrome. The infection may occur several weeks before the development of the arthritis, the urethritis, and the conjunctivitis, and the infections seem to fall into two broad categories:

those from venereal exposure and those related to diarrhea. In the United States there is usually a sexual exposure to the disease shortly before the development of discharge from the penis, which is usually the first symptom. Reiter's syndrome is not considered a definite venereal disease, but most physicians think venereal exposure to be a likely cause in many cases. The infection appears to cause Reiter's syndrome in those susceptible individuals with the B27 gene.

Another form of this syndrome follows episodes of diarrhea. This form can occur in epidemics and is most frequently related to *shigella dysentery,* a form of bacterial diarrhea. Several well-studied epidemics suggest that about 20% of subjects who are B27, positive and experience shigella dysentery will develop Reiter's syndrome.

It seems likely that no single bacterium causes all cases. The *Shigella* infection is the best established, but some of the venereal cases appear to follow infection with organisms called *Chlamydia* or *Mycoplasma.* Somewhat similar problems are seen after infection with *Yersinia* or *Salmonella* organisms. Thus, different infectious syndromes may precede development of Reiter's syndrome.

This interplay between the genetic predisposition represented by the B27 gene and the necessity for attack by a microorganism provides a fascinating interaction for scientific study. These studies, now being conducted at many medical centers, are likely to lead to major advances in managing Reiter's syndrome.

FEATURES

Reiter's syndrome occurs mostly in men and is usually episodic, with each episode lasting several weeks to several months. It frequently recurs in subsequent years, and it shares many features with ankylosing spondylitis and psoriatic arthritis.

As with ankylosing spondylitis, the main problem is at the attachment where ligaments and tendons insert into the bone. Thus, involvement of the sacroiliac joints and of the spine is common. Since Reiter's syndrome tends to involve the peripheral parts of the body more than ankylosing spondylitis, a common feature is heel pain, either on the bottom of the heel where the ligaments that form the arch attach or on the back of the heel where the Achilles tendon attaches.

Like psoriatic arthritis, Reiter's syndrome tends to involve the peripheral joints in a random way. Thus, just a few joints are usually involved, and these joints are usually not the same on the two sides of the body. Reiter's syndrome frequently involves one side of the body while sparing the other, and it may skip around from one side to the other in different parts of the spine. A "sausage digit," as described on page 31, is sometimes seen. In psoriatic arthritis, the upper extremities usually are involved more than the lower, while with Reiter's syndrome the feet and toes are more frequently involved than are the hands.

Eye problems usually involve only one eye at a time. This may be conjunctivitis ("pink eye") or an inflammation affecting the deeper parts of the eye, causing pain on exposure to bright light or interference with vision.

Discharge from the penis is the third major feature and usually consists of a clear, watery discharge that does not cause discomfort. While this frequently lasts only a few days or weeks, it may reappear later.

A skin rash occurs in only a few patients, but it can help with the diagnosis. The scaling red skin lesions are most common on the palms and soles and are sometimes not immediately noticed because they don't hurt or itch. Shallow sores of the penis or of the female genital organs may occur; these are also usually painless. Some cases of Reiter's syndrome with skin involvement resemble psoriatic arthritis, and distinction between the two can be difficult.

Tests

X-ray changes usually take several years to develop. Inflammation of the sacroiliac joint, as in ankylosing spondylitis, is common. Stiffening of the spine can also be seen. X-rays of the heels may show bone spurs at the points of attachment where the heel pain is noted.

Laboratory tests are not particularly helpful in diagnosis. The latex test for rheumatoid factor is negative. The antinuclear antibody test is negative. The sedimentation rate is sometimes elevated and sometimes not. The test for the B27 antigen will be positive about 70% of the time.

PROGNOSIS

Reiter's syndrome is characterized by an episodic course. Some patients have only one episode and no recurrences. For others, periods of activity of the disease will alternate with periods of relative inactivity. It is unusual for the arthritis to be severely crippling, but this can happen.

In a very few cases, problems with the eye can result in loss of sight, usually in just one eye and late in the disease. The skin problems seldom pose real difficulties and are usually present only a small part of the time.

Those individuals with Reiter's syndrome who do not have the B27 gene probably do a little better than those who have the gene. The first episode usually gives some indication of the disease's future severity. Like most forms of arthritis, Reiter's syndrome varies from mild to severe, with most patients doing quite well.

TREATMENT

As in ankylosing spondylitis, the most frequent medications used are indomethacin (p. 124) and naproxen (p. 128). In very severe cases, methotrexate (p. 150), azathioprine (p. 151), or experimental drugs may be required. Corticosteroids such as prednisone are not very helpful and should almost never be used.

Reiter's syndrome is sometimes difficult to treat and may be resistant to all of the anti-inflammatory agents. Sometimes a drug that seemed ineffective when first used will prove effective when used again a few weeks or even months later. Hence, when the disease is difficult to control the physician may periodically rotate drugs to determine which will work the best. Since the disease comes in cycles control can ultimately be achieved, but it may take disturbingly long to find the right treatment.

Although infections seem to cause Reiter's syndrome antibiotics do not seem to be an effective treatment. Many physicians have tried tetracycline and other antibiotics, but the results have been inconsistent.

Eye involvement may require treatment with corticosteroids applied locally. In severe cases the steroid may be injected into the eye or behind the eye. The skin problems seldom require any treatment. Involvement of the aortic valve, exceedingly rare, may require replacement of that valve surgically.

Surgery for the joints is rarely needed in Reiter's syndrome. Range-of-motion exercises and a judicious balance between rest and graded exercise are important. See instructions for particular joints in Part III.

If you have Reiter's syndrome, proceed to Part II, page 103.

CHAPTER 5

Crystal Arthritis

Inflammation Within the Joint Space

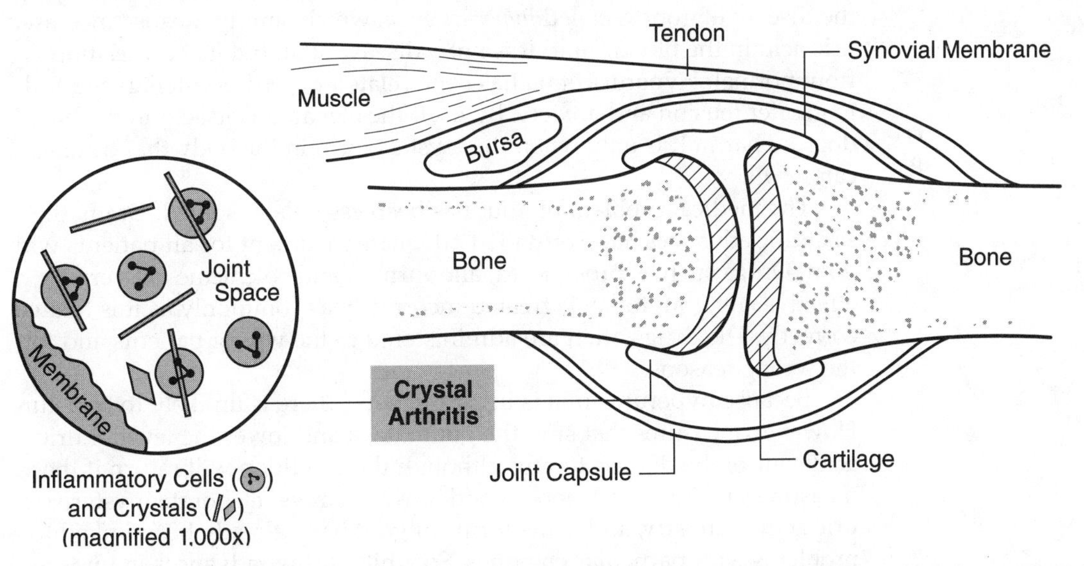

In crystal (or microcrystalline) arthritis, chemical crystals in the joint space cause an inflammation to develop. The inflammation represents the efforts of the body to remove the crystals, but the process is very painful. Gout and pseudogout are the two most common kinds of crystal arthritis.

Gout

The term gout calls to mind a king, rather red-faced and corpulent, reclining in an easy chair with a very sore foot propped up on a pillow. In fact, gout is a most painful disease and can sometimes result from overindulgence. Many people don't think that gout is arthritis, but it most certainly is. It is the best example of a crystal arthritis, in which the body's reaction to small mineral crystals in the joint space causes a painful illness. The crystals of gout are made up of uric acid, and the inflammatory reaction is extremely intense.

Gout crystals cannot develop without an elevated level of uric acid in the body fluids. Unless the level is high in the fluid in the joint, no crystals can form and no reaction can take place. Hence, the condition underlying the disease of gout is called *hyperuricemia,* which simply means "increased uric acid in the blood," and it is not a disease at all but just a variation from normal. Hyperuricemia has been related to greater intelligence and to greater tension and anxiety. By itself the elevated uric acid in the blood does no harm. It is only when the crystals form in the body that trouble can result.

The medical problem of gout has been essentially solved. Dramatic scientific advances have provided adequate treatment for all patients with gout. Drugs such as probenecid, allopurinol, and colchicine are very effective. Yet gout today is treated incorrectly as commonly as it is treated correctly. The drugs often are administered to the wrong patients and for the wrong reasons.

Because hyperuricemia is in part genetic, there is unlikely to be a cure. However, measures that stop the gout attack and lower the level of uric acid control the disease totally, although the condition will return if these measures are stopped. Science continues to unravel elaborate mysteries of uric acid chemistry, and some forms of gout have already been linked to problems with particular enzymes. So while further advances in understanding the disease are likely, the therapy of today is entirely satisfactory and is not likely to be improved within the foreseeable future.

FEATURES

Gout consists of four stages, beginning with the tendency to develop gout and progressing through the gouty attack to a long-term disease. Many people have the first stage and very few experience the last.

The first stage is called *asymptomatic hyperuricemia.* This means that the level of uric acid in the blood is raised without any resulting problems. Uric acid levels go up a little in boys at about puberty and in women at about the time of menopause, so sex hormones have some effect on uric acid level. The levels will go up before an examination at school or at a particularly stressful time of life. Asymptomatic hyperuricemia is defined as having a uric acid level higher than that of 95% of the population. With most tests used today, this means a level higher than about 8 mg per hundred mg. Asymptomatic hyperuricemia fluctuates somewhat, but it tends to persist once it has occurred. Even in those few subjects who go on to the second stage, the period of asymptomatic hyperuricemia usually lasts about 20 years before anything happens.

Acute gouty arthritis, or gout, is the second stage. Here the body fluids saturated with uric acid have begun to form crystals. The crystals form in the joint fluid, and the body reacts with a strong inflammatory reaction. Sometimes there is no apparent cause for the attack of gout; other times it happens after surgery, after eating particularly rich foods, after an alcoholic binge, or after an injury to the area. At any rate, the affected part begins to swell and becomes red and painful over a period of a few hours. Soon the area is too tender to touch; even the touch of bedclothes causes exquisite pain. If not treated the attack will peak in two or three days and will gradually disappear over about a two-week period. After the attack the joint and surrounding tissue are entirely normal until the next attack.

Acute gout affects most commonly the base of the big toe. This form of gout is so common as to have a special name, *podagra.* Next most common is the knee, then the ankle, and then the instep of the foot. Less frequently joints of the upper extremity, particularly the shoulder, wrist, or elbow, may be involved. As a rule, just one joint is involved at a time. Very rarely, two, three, or four joints are involved simultaneously—never more. Patients with a strong tendency toward gout may have five or six attacks a year.

The third, rather simple stage is called *interval gout.* This is the same as the first stage, except that it represents the period between attacks in a patient who has already had an attack of gout. During this stage asymptomatic hyperuricemia is present, but the likelihood of an attack of gout is much greater for the patient who has previously had an attack.

The fourth stage is called *chronic tophaceous gout.* This problem, unlike acute gout, does not come and go. Here the crystals of uric acid have begun to accumulate in the body, causing deposits of a gritty, chalky material. These deposits are called *tophi.* They can sometimes be seen just under the skin, particularly around the joints and in the ear. They can also grow inside the bone near the joints, causing destruction of the bone. In rare circumstances they form inside the kidney and can interfere with kidney function. Kidney stones composed of the uric acid sometimes form. Fortunately, because of advances in treatment, this fourth stage of disease is now seldom seen.

Doctors generally think of gout as occurring in two types of patients. In the first type, the body makes too much uric acid; the kidneys excrete the uric acid normally into the urine but can't get rid of it fast enough. In the second type, the body makes a normal amount of uric acid but the kidneys are unable to get rid of it adequately, so the blood level increases. The first type of gout, with increased production of uric acid, is the more serious and can lead to the problems of tophaceous gout.

Tests

The uric acid test can be important to diagnosis; however, as this test is sometimes inaccurate, a doctor may wish to repeat it with another version (called the *uricase* method) that gives a more accurate result. Many doctors will want to measure the amount of uric acid in a 24-hour urine specimen (p. 174) to determine how much uric acid the body is excreting.

Acute gout is one of a few diseases that can be diagnosed absolutely accurately. This is done by taking a sample of the joint fluid and looking at it under the microscope. In 95% of acute gout cases the uric acid crystals can be seen in the joint fluid, surrounded by the body's white cells, which are trying frantically to eat them. The crystals can be seen clearly only with polarized light, so polarizing lenses are required for the microscope.

PROGNOSIS

The overall prognosis for gout is always excellent. No significant problem with health should result from a gouty condition if the patient carefully follows the recommendations of a competent physician. The prognosis varies depending on the stage of the disease.

Asymptomatic hyperuricemia is not a disease at all and very seldom requires treatment. The prognosis does depend on the level of the elevated uric acid; patients with uric acid levels in the very highest ranges have at least a 50% chance of developing an attack of gout or of developing a kidney stone. The exact frequency of acute gout or kidney stone is still debated, but it is infrequent except at very high levels of uric acid.

Acute gout will run its course, without treatment, over a couple of weeks. However, with treatment, relief can usually be obtained in just a few hours and the response to treatment is usually dramatic. Thus, acute gout requires treatment as soon as possible in the course of the attack.

During the interval between attacks, the frequency of previous attacks is the best guide to their recurrence. After a single first attack, only half of patients will have a second. Thereafter, recurrence becomes the rule rather than the exception. These additional attacks usually can be prevented by appropriate treatment.

In tophaceous gout, stage four, the condition slowly progresses until some damage is caused to the joints or the kidneys. With treatment the tophi slowly dissolve and are excreted through the urine as uric acid. If the tophi are large, they may leave some destruction behind, but usually there is healing. Hence, while we don't like to see tophaceous gout (and see it very rarely now), even this stage can be effectively treated.

There is still controversy about the effects of elevated levels of uric acid on the kidney. Theoretically damage could occur, but in practice we can't detect any significant problem. Any kidney disease due to uric acid would progress very slowly over a period of years and should be easily treatable until very advanced. Hence, most doctors feel that kidney tests should be performed every few years in patients with elevated uric acid levels but that treatment is not required in the absence of an actual problem.

TREATMENT

For some patients gout is a disease of lifestyle. It is affected by body weight, diet, and alcohol. Thus, it can be treated by a more rational lifestyle, including a reasonable body weight, a good exercise level, and a diet that excludes foods high in uric acid, such as liver, pancreas, and brain. Strict diets are very seldom needed. Intake of a large amount of fluid will increase urine flow and assist in removing uric acid from the body. Making the urine more basic, as by taking sodium bicarbonate (baking soda), will result in faster elimination of uric acid, since uric acid is more soluble when the urine is alkaline (basic) than when it is acid.

Moreover, a lot of problems associated with elevated uric acid levels are caused by drugs, and stopping those drugs or switching to less bothersome ones can alleviate the problem entirely. Most notorious are water pills or diuretics (particularly the thiazide diuretics such as Diuril or Dyazide), but many other drugs also can cause elevation of uric acid. This is just another reason to manage your life with as few drugs as possible.

Medical treatment is the mainstay of managing gout. Selection of the particular drug depends on the stage of the disease. With asymptomatic hyperuricemia no treatment is required, and you should question a treatment recommendation if you are not having problems. To be rational at all, treatment of an elevated uric acid level must be continued for life, and in a typical American patient with treatment begun at age 35, the cost and compound interest on the drugs used may exceed $40,000! The treatment will involve 38,325 pills! For most people, any value received from such treatment will not justify its cost, and some patients will experience side effects that will increase the cost yet more.

Acute gout is treated with agents that block the inflammatory reaction, and a number of drugs do this effectively. Colchicine, the traditional favorite, can be given by mouth or by vein. Its problem: it causes diarrhea when given by mouth, and the diarrhea can be quite severe. Indomethacin (p. 124) and other anti-inflammatory agents are frequently effective. And ACTH injections or corticosteroids are favored by a few physicians, although not by most. Any of these may be used; patients who have compared several different treatments tend to prefer colchicine by vein.

In the interval between attacks, a drug may be given to reduce the uric acid level. Usually these agents are not started during the attack because they can prolong the acute attack. Probenecid and allopurinol are the two most frequent choices; probenecid is usually preferred unless the 24-hour urine test shows excretion of a large amount of uric acid, in which case allopurinol is often chosen. With both of these drugs, low-dose colchicine is also frequently used to prevent attacks. The colchicine dose can be low enough that diarrhea does not occur, and it is effective in reducing the number of new attacks. Meanwhile the excess uric acid in the body is being slowly eliminated through the urine.

With chronic tophaceous gout (stage four), an agent to increase excretion or decrease production of uric acid is essential. Probenecid or allopurinol should always be used. Colchicine also may be used to limit the frequency of acute attacks. In severe cases probenecid and allopurinol may be used together. Because of effective treatment, chronic tophaceous gout is a vanishing disease. Ask your doctor about drugs for gout.

If your problem is gout, proceed to Part II, page 103.

Pseudogout

The colorful and apt name of this condition suggests that the disease is similar to gout, as is the case, and *pseudogout* is a much less cumbersome term than the alternative names, *calcium pyrophosphate crystal deposition disease* and *chondrocalcinosis.* As in gout, crystals in the joint space cause an intense inflammatory reaction that results in redness and pain in the joint. In pseudogout, the crystals are not uric acid but are pyrophosphate crystals. They do not form in the joint space but are deposited there from the nearby cartilage, where they can be seen on an X-ray. *Chondro* means "cartilage"; hence the name *chondrocalcinosis* refers to calcium in the cartilage of the joint. A similar syndrome occurs with other minerals that can form crystals, such as hydroxyapatite, but uric acid and calcium pyrophosphate are the two main offenders. The calcium does not come from drinking too much milk, and diet will neither help nor hurt this condition.

Pseudogout is much more a disease of aging than is gout, and the calcium accumulates slowly in the cartilage over a long period. In patients with rare metabolic diseases, such as parathyroid disease or hemochromatosis, the condition may occur earlier in life. Generally, however, pseudogout is a disease of the later years.

FEATURES

Typically, a patient with pseudogout will have acute attacks of crystal arthritis much like gout. The calcium crystals excite a less violent response than do uric acid crystals, so pain is not always as severe, but the discharge of crystals may last longer, causing the attack to last longer. Hence, many patients with pseudogout don't have as clear a pattern of attacks separated by symptom-free intervals. They may have problems more or less continuously.

The average age of a patient at first attack is about 70 years. Men and women are affected in approximately similar frequencies (unlike gout, which tends to affect men more frequently than women). The joint most often involved is the knee, followed by the wrists and the ankles. More often than in gout, several joints may be involved at one time. Attacks may be brought on by stress or surgery, as with gout, but overeating or the eating of rich foods is not related to attacks.

Often there is some cartilage degeneration (osteoarthrosis) in the affected joints, and the tendency of this condition to last for weeks or months may be partly related to the associated osteoarthrosis.

Tests

Laboratory tests are not very helpful. Blood tests are usually entirely normal. But X-ray findings are very important. On the X-ray, calcium can be seen in the cartilage of the affected joints and sometimes in other joints. And if the joint fluid is removed through a needle, the crystals of calcium pyrophosphate can be seen in the joint fluid. These rather square crystals contrast with the long, needlelike crystals seen in gout.

Together, the finding of calcium in the cartilage on X-ray and the identification of calcium crystals in the joint fluid establish the diagnosis of pseudogout.

PROGNOSIS

The prognosis for pseudogout is good. Very seldom does crippling result, although over half of pseudogout patients will have recurrent attacks and many will experience some degree of sustained pain. Attacks may continue for a long time. Patients tend to get better for a while and then worse for a while; most patients are able to carry on quite normal activities despite the problems.

Pseudogout seems to affect only the joints, so patients feel entirely well otherwise. There is no involvement of other organs and, thus, no truly serious threats to health. The condition does not seem to be genetically influenced so there is no particular risk to family members.

TREATMENT

Treatment is helpful but not as dramatically so as with gout. The most effective drugs are indomethacin (p. 124) or other nonsteroidal anti-inflammatory agents. Frequently these agents must be taken rather steadily to continue the relief. Colchicine, which is consistently effective in gout, helps some people with pseudogout, but does not seem to help others.

Careful exercises and graded activities for the involved joints and preservation of a normal lifestyle are important. (See the discussions in Part III for specific instructions.) Weight control is particularly crucial if the weight-bearing joints are affected by the pseudogout. Techniques of joint protection, as described in Part III, pages 212–239, are helpful.

The drugs for gout that control uric acid level, such as allopurinol and probenecid, would not be expected to work in pseudogout, and they don't. The uric acid level is normal in pseudogout. Surgery is very seldom required, but we have seen patients who eventually needed replacement of a knee or even a hip. In general, treatment should be mild and conservative. Strong agents such as cortisone and its derivatives are not helpful and carry serious hazards, although corticosteroid injections into the joint are sometimes helpful.

If your problem is pseudogout, proceed to Part II, page 103.

CHAPTER 6

Infections

Infection of the Joint Space

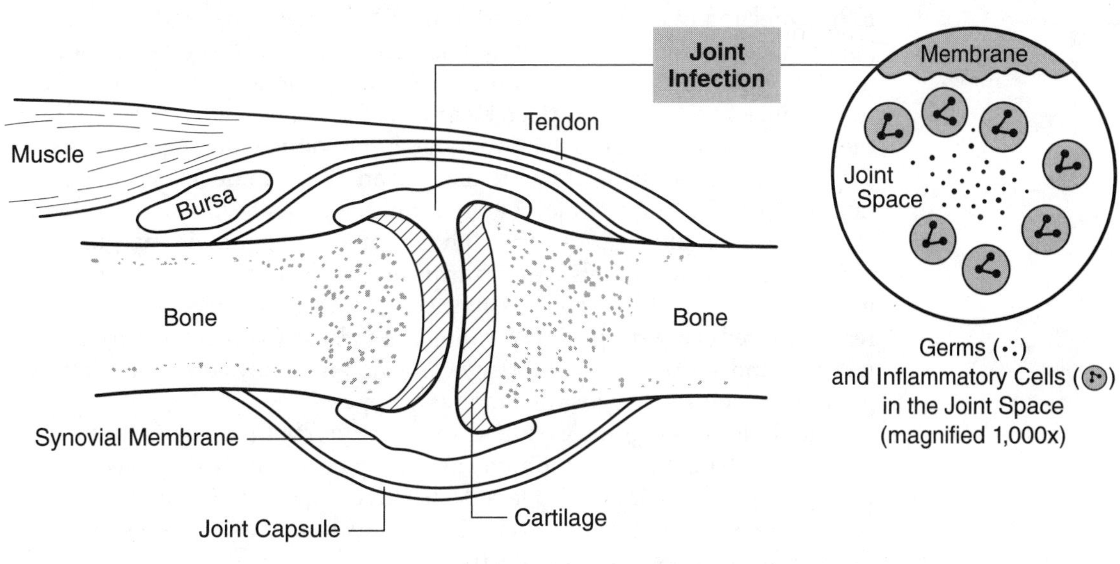

Germs (•:) and Inflammatory Cells in the Joint Space (magnified 1,000x)

If bacteria lodge and grow within the joint space, an "infectious" arthritis is present. This kind of arthritis requires antibiotics, and treatment represents an emergency. The infection can spread to other parts of the body or can destroy the involved joint.

The most common bacteria causing this problem are the **Staphylococcus,** the **Gonococcus,** and the tuberculosis germ. Lyme disease is a somewhat similar condition.

Staphylococcus *(Staph)*

The "single hot joint" is an emergency and needs immediate attention because it might be a bacterial infection. When bacteria invade the joint space, the joint becomes a giant boil filled with pus. Warm, red skin surrounds the joint, and there is swelling with considerable pain.

Almost every type of bacterium seems at some time or another to have caused an infectious arthritis, but *Staphylococcus* and *Gonococcus* (discussed in the next section) infections are the two most common. The *Staphylococcus* infection is possibly the most serious. Arthritis problems due to these or any other bacteria are all treated similarly.

How do bacteria get into the joint? Sometimes they get in through the bloodstream as part of an infection elsewhere in the body. Sometimes the initial infection may not be noticed, but a few bacteria may lodge in the joint while passing by. More rarely, bacteria are introduced by a previous injection into the knee or by a direct injury. Infection is a rare complication of joint injection and can happen even with the most careful physician and the best techniques. Germs tend to lodge in previously damaged joints, so patients with arthritis are more likely than others to develop an infectious arthritis. A single hot joint appearing in a patient with an underlying arthritis is even more serious than a hot joint in a patient with no previous arthritis. Some individuals with arthritis are more susceptible to joint infection because of lowered resistance due to a serious disease or resistance-reducing drugs. Intravenous drug abuse (usually heroin) is a frequent and serious cause. In many cases no one knows how the bacteria got into the joint—they just mysteriously appear.

Staphylococcal germs vary, and some are worse than others. With a particularly bad strain of staph, the joint may be seriously damaged in as little as one or two days; with less destructive organisms it may take several weeks for damage to occur. Staph infection of a joint is a serious disease that can result in joint destruction.

FEATURES

Bacterial infection of the joint, with *Staphylococcus* as the best example, develops over a period of hours to days. The arthritis is severe and the affected joint is red, warm, and swollen. A staphylococcal infection of a joint is in no way subtle; symptoms are pronounced and the signs are usually obvious.

Usually only one joint is involved, although on occasion two or three or even four may be involved. Infections tend to occur in the largest joints of the body. The knee is the joint most frequently infected. Infection is also relatively common in the ankle, the wrist, the shoulder, the elbow, and the hips. Other joints are affected less frequently.

Tests

Since this is an infection, there may be fever and the patient may feel generally ill. The white blood count may be elevated and the sedimentation rate may be raised. Both of these tests may be normal in some cases. Other blood tests are not helpful, except for a culture of the blood, which is used to identify the offending bacterium.

X-rays may show bone destruction at the joint after a few days or a few months, if treatment was not begun early enough. The changes revealed by X-ray lag behind the disease's progress, however, so the X-ray is not as helpful as might be supposed.

The key test is removal of fluid from the joint, examination of this fluid under the microscope, and culture of the fluid for bacteria. The joint fluid will look like pus and will be swarming with polymorphonuclear white cells trying to fight the infection. The bacteria will be seen in the joint fluid and sometimes inside the cells that are trying to engulf them. The culture, available one to two days later, will usually permit a positive identification. The joint fluid test also allows the doctor to eliminate the possibility of gout, which is the most frequently confused diagnosis.

PROGNOSIS

Staphylococcal infection of the joint, if identified and treated properly, has an excellent prognosis. In two weeks the joint should be much better, although fluid may accumulate for yet another week or so. There should be no long-term bad results of any kind. If treatment is delayed, destruction of the bone and seeding of the infection to other parts of the body may occur, with ominous consequences. Without any treatment, staphylococcal joint infection would be a fatal disease most of the time.

Relatively rarely, the bone next to the joint may become infected (osteomyelitis). This can be a serious complication requiring long-term antibiotic treatment or surgery.

TREATMENT

A high "index of suspicion" and a prompt diagnosis are the keys to good results in treating staph infections. The proper antibiotics must be started as quickly as possible and in adequate doses. Except in patients who are allergic to penicillin, one of the penicillinlike antibiotics will be used. Initial treatment is by intravenous infusion, and almost all doctors hospitalize patients with staphylococcal joint infections, at least during the early stages of treatment. If a great deal of fluid is accumulating it may be removed from the joint with a needle every day or every several days. If this is still not adequate, surgical drainage of the extra pus is performed by some physicians. The antibiotic should be continued for at least ten days to two weeks, and often for six weeks. Some follow-up is needed to ensure that the infection is gone and that there is no related infection in the bone.

This form of arthritis can be cured—or it can be fatal. Cure requires that you consult a competent physician promptly so that appropriate treatment may be started. The single hot joint is a signal to see the physician today.

If your problem is staphylococcal arthritis, proceed to Part II, page 103.

Gonococcus *(GC)*

We think of gonorrhea as a venereal disease. Sometimes it is called GC, or clap, or the whites, or some other picturesque name. It is less well known that gonorrhea can cause an arthritis called *gonococcal arthritis.* This is an infectious arthritis in which the gonococcal bacteria grow in the joint space. This is one of the most common causes of arthritis in young women between the ages of 15 and 25.

During a genital infection with gonococcal bacteria, the bacteria may travel in the blood to the joint space. Gonococcal bacteria are unusual in that they grow well only in particular parts of the body, such as the urethra or the joints. The body defenses are good against the GC organism; even bloodstream infections that have seeded the joints can occasionally be overcome by body defenses alone, without the aid of antibiotics, although, of course, this is not desirable.

FEATURES

For the most part, gonococcal arthritis is a disease of young women. It occurs ten times as frequently in women as in men. There appear to be several reasons for this. In women the gonorrhea infection of the vagina and cervix may not be noticed by the patient, whereas a man almost always notices discharge from the penis. So in women the infection may remain untreated until a menstrual period comes. During the menstrual period the bacteria can get into the bloodstream from the uterus and can move through the bloodstream to other areas of the body. Most cases of gonococcal arthritis begin during the menstrual period.

Gonococcal arthritis affects one to several joints but does not affect many joints at the same time. The most common joint is the knee. Second most common is the wrist, with a tendency to involve the back of the wrist around the tendons that operate the fingers. This is called *tenosynovitis.* The arthritis caused by gonococcal infection will seem to move from one joint to another and usually will not be the same on both sides of the body. For example, a right knee, a left wrist, and a right ankle may be affected.

The skin can provide important clues to the presence of a gonococcal infection. Little blisters on a red base may be found, often only one or two over the entire body. These blisters contain the gonococcal bacteria and are evidence that the infection has moved through the bloodstream and might be infecting the joints.

In men, a white or slightly yellowish discharge from the penis is almost always present. In women, a vaginal discharge and sometimes fever or abdominal pain may be present. Infection of the rectum or of the mouth may occur with the gonococcal bacteria.

Tests

Physicians will usually culture the various body fluids that may be infected to identify the bacteria. The discharge from the penis or the vagina is usually culture positive, but a culture from the joint fluid is frequently negative. This may indicate that the body is already in the process of cleaning up that infection.

No other laboratory findings are positive, with the exception of an elevated white count indicating infection, or perhaps a mildly elevated sedimentation rate. There usually will not be any X-ray changes.

PROGNOSIS

Gonococcal arthritis clears up without any damage if it is diagnosed promptly and treated properly. It may take several days to get the joints all calmed down, and fluid may reaccumulate in some joints for several weeks, but ultimately all symptoms clear up and there are no residual problems unless the patient is reinfected.

Even before antibiotic treatment was available, most people did not suffer disability from gonococcal arthritis. However, with the potential for serious complications and with curative treatment available, it is essential that all patients be promptly diagnosed and treated.

TREATMENT

The key to treatment is antibiotics. Usually the antibiotic will be penicillin or one of its derivatives (unless the patient is allergic to penicillin). Many physicians hospitalize the patient for the first few days and may administer the antibiotics through the vein to ensure that the antibiotic directly attacks the bacteria site. On some occasions the joint will be drained of excess fluid, and in rare instances antibiotics may be put directly into an infected joint. Usually this is not necessary.

It must be remembered that gonococcal arthritis comes from a venereal disease. Treatment includes not only the patient but also the sexual contacts of the patient, who may be unknowingly spreading the disease to additional persons. If you are the patient, it is critical that you help your sexual partners by ensuring that they know about the disease and that they go for adequate treatment. Help is readily available at the local health department.

If your problem is gonococcal arthritis, proceed to Part II, page 103.

Tuberculosis (TB)

Tuberculosis of the joint is rare. For that matter, tuberculosis itself is relatively rare, even though it is now increasing in frequency. But arthritis caused by a tuberculosis bacterium is typical of slow, less obvious infections of the joint space, so we describe it here. Not only the tuberculosis bacterium but also various kinds of fungi, such as histoplasmosis or coccidioidomycosis, may result in the same sort of slow, long-term joint infection.

As many as 50% of patients with arthritis due to tuberculosis do not have tuberculosis of the lungs. Tuberculous arthritis may develop for months or even years before a diagnosis is made. Treatment of the joint problem is usually not difficult, but because the condition is rare neither doctor nor patient may think of it.

Don't worry too much about having tuberculosis of a joint, because it is very unusual. But bear in mind that a long-term "cold" swelling of a single joint occasionally may be due to an infection, just like the short-term, red, "hot" process that we usually associate with infection.

FEATURES

In one study, tuberculous arthritis was not diagnosed for an average of 19 months, and in one patient the process of making the diagnosis took 12 years.

Usually the knee or the hip is involved. The tuberculosis organism needs a large space to grow in, so the smaller joints are generally not infected; once in a while we will see arthritis caused by tuberculosis or a fungus in the small joint of the hand or foot. Usually just one joint is involved. Arthritis is seen in far less than 1% of patients with tuberculosis.

Tuberculosis of the spine used to be called Pott's disease. It was fairly common at one time, although in recent years cases have been few and far between. The key feature of a Pott's abscess (or of a tuberculous arthritis of a knee or wrist) is that it is a "cold" abscess. Unlike bacterial infections (for example, boils), tuberculosis and fungus do not excite a very violent inflammation, and the affected area is usually about the same temperature as the surrounding tissues instead of being hot and red.

Tests

Diagnosis can be made by culture of the joint fluid in 80% of cases. A biopsy of the lining tissue of the joint, the synovium, will be positive in most of the rest. Some scientists have thought that a low glucose (blood sugar) in the synovial space is common in tuberculous arthritis; others have found this less frequently.

X-rays taken over a long period may show some destruction of the bone next to the joint infection. The bone changes usually take years to develop, and it is unlikely that any will be present until after a number of months have passed.

Laboratory tests commonly positive in other forms of arthritis will usually be negative in tuberculous arthritis.

PROGNOSIS

In tuberculous arthritis prognosis depends on the time of diagnosis. If the diagnosis is early and the tuberculosis in other parts of the body is not causing major problems, the prognosis is for complete recovery. The tuberculous infection can be cured and the patient will have no disability. If diagnosis is delayed and there has been destruction of the cartilage, then there may be some disability. Occasionally, in the presence of severe tuberculosis in other parts of the body, not even good treatment will prevent death.

TREATMENT

Suspicion of the disease and the making of a correct diagnosis are crucial. After diagnosis the joint fluid may be drained periodically. Antituberculosis medications are given by mouth for two to three years. Improvement is generally noted within the first few weeks and is complete within a few months. Treatment is continued longer than this to prevent recurrence.

If your problem is tuberculous arthritis, proceed to Part II, page 103.

Lyme Disease

A skin disease related to tick bites, *erythema chronicum migricans,* has been recognized in northern Europe for many decades. Only in the last two decades has the disease been discovered in the United States and its basis understood. A cluster of cases, many of them in children, discovered in and around the town of Old Lyme, Connecticut, drew attention to the condition and gave Lyme disease its name.

The disease is caused by a bacterial spirochete, *Borrelia burgdorferi,* which infects a certain strain of ticks and is transmitted to humans by a bite from an infected tick. Only a bite from an infected tick can result in the disease, and the infection is found only in some geographical areas. In Connecticut and Long Island, New York, many ticks are infected. In northern California, a few are; in most other locations, very few. This is a deer tick, and deer serve as the reservoir for the disease.

FEATURES

At the site of the tick bite a rather round red skin rash may appear and expand, often to the size of a hand or even larger. Other red spots, usually smaller, may appear elsewhere on the body. Some people either don't recognize the rash or don't have it, and many don't remember receiving the tick bite although they recently walked through woods or fields. Usually the tick must remain in place for a day or so for Lyme disease to develop.

A few days or weeks after the bite other symptoms may develop, including arthritis and neurological disease such as paralysis of one or more nerves. The arthritis is variable; it may involve one joint or many, and it may be present for a brief period or for years. In some patients it can resemble rheumatoid arthritis.

PROGNOSIS

Generally prognosis is good but variable. It is likely that *Lyme disease* is greatly overdiagnosed today. The term has been widely used in the popular press and many patients come to their doctors asking for an unnecessary blood test for Lyme disease. Unfortunately, this test for antibodies to the spirochete is not very good, and it often indicates "borderline positive" for healthy people who have not had tick bites. If you do not live in a community where Lyme disease is common, the chance that your arthritis was caused by the Lyme spirochete is remote.

TREATMENT

The infection can be effectively treated with antibiotics such as penicillin or tetracycline, but only in the first few days of the illness. Certainly all patients showing the migrating red skin spots should be treated. Most doctors will also try a course of antibiotics later on, but it usually doesn't work then. If you have Lyme disease be sure that your doctor knows all about the disease since new treatments are likely to be developed as our knowledge of the condition increases.

If your problem is Lyme disease, proceed to Part II, page 103.

Viral Infections

The joints can be affected by other infectious agents, including viruses. These problems are minor, unusual, and last only a few days or weeks. German measles (rubella) can cause such a reaction, as can immunization against German measles. Hepatitis can do the same.

If your problem is viral arthritis, proceed to Part II, page 103

CHAPTER 7

Cartilage Degeneration

Thinning of the Joint Gristle

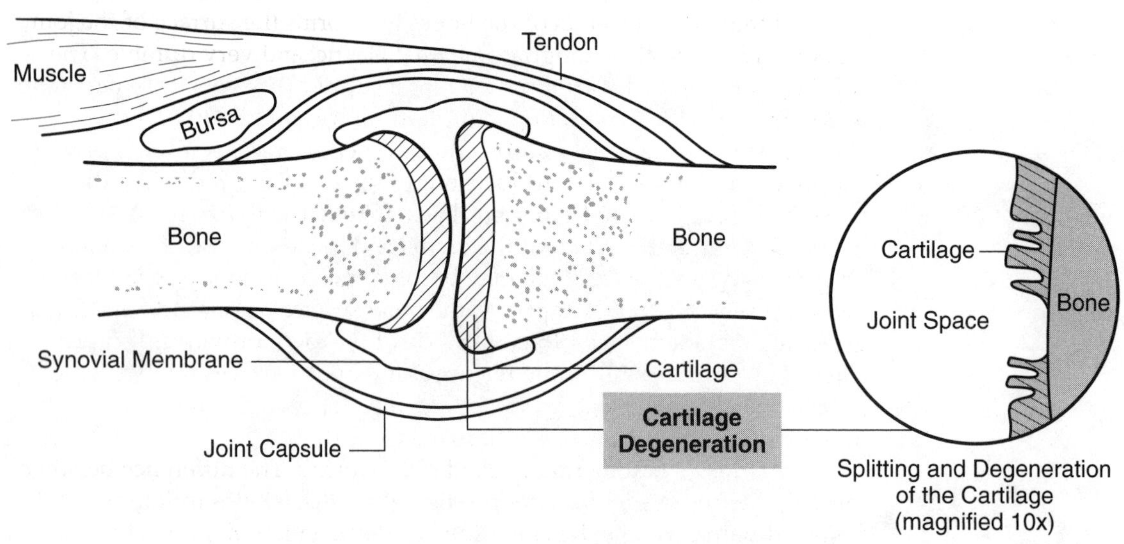

The cartilage, or gristle, which absorbs the shock of joint motion, can become thin and degenerate, leaving two surfaces of bone in contact with one another. The cartilage first frays and splits, and eventually can almost disappear. There is little or no inflammation. This type of arthritis is called osteoarthritis, OA, degenerative joint disease, DJD, or osteoarthrosis.

Osteoarthritis (Osteoarthrosis, OA, Degenerative Joint Disease, DJD)

This is the kind of arthritis that almost everybody gets eventually—a practically universal problem that increases with age. It is not as responsive to medical treatment as we might like. Fortunately osteoarthritis is usually a mild condition. The majority of people with osteoarthritis don't have any pain or stiffness, and the majority of the remainder have only occasional problems. Hence, osteoarthritis usually is a much more benign form of arthritis than those discussed previously. In other words, the changes in the skeleton that occur with age are inevitable, but they cause symptoms in relatively few people and severe symptoms in even fewer.

The tissue involved in osteoarthritis is the cartilage. This is the gristle material that faces the ends of the bones and forms the surface of the joint on both sides. Gristle is tough, somewhat elastic, and very durable. The cartilage, or gristle, does not have a blood supply, so it gets its oxygen and nutrition from the surrounding joint fluid. In this it is aided by being elastic and by being able to absorb fluid. When we use a joint, the pressure expresses fluid and waste products out of the cartilage, and when the pressure is relieved, the fluid seeps back, together with oxygen and nutrients. Hence, the health of the cartilage depends on use of the joint. Over many years the cartilage may become frayed and may even wear away entirely. When this happens, the bone surface on one side of the joint grates against the bone on the other side of the joint, providing a much less elastic joint surface. With time the opposing bony surfaces may become polished, a process called *eburnation.* As this happens the joint may again move more smoothly and cause less discomfort.

Osteoarthritis is sometimes called *osteoarthrosis.* The difference between these two terms has to do with inflammation. *Itis* denotes inflammation, and with cartilage degeneration very little inflammation is found. Hence, some experts prefer the term *osteoarthrosis,* which does not imply inflammation.

There are three common forms of osteoarthritis, and many people have some of each type. The first and mildest causes knobby enlargement of the finger joints. The end joints of the fingers become bony and the hands begin to assume the appearance we associate with old age. The other joints of the fingers also may be involved. The joint at the base of the thumb is often affected. This kind of arthritis (or arthrosis) usually causes little difficulty beyond the cosmetic. There may be some stiffness.

The second form of osteoarthritis involves the spine, specifically the disks between vertebrae. Bony growths appear on the spinal disks in the neck region or in the low back. Usually the bony growths are associated with some narrowing of the space between the vertebrae. Disks, not cartilage, become frayed in this condition. Changes in the spine begin early in life in almost all of us, but cause symptoms relatively seldom.

The third form of osteoarthritis involves the weight-bearing joints, almost always the hips and knees. These problems can be quite severe.

It is possible to have all three kinds of osteoarthrosis or any two of them, but often a patient will have only one.

Patients who have had fractures near a joint or have a congenital malformation at a joint seem to develop osteoarthritis in those joints at an earlier age. On the other hand, the usual description of this arthritis as "wear and tear" is not accurate. While excessive wear and tear on the joint can theoretically result in damage, activity also helps the joint remain supple and lubricated, and this tends to cancel out the theoretical bad effects.

At any rate, careful studies of people who regularly put a lot of stress on joints (such as individuals who operate pneumatic drills or run long distances on hard paved surfaces) have been unable to establish a relationship between these activities and the development of arthritis. Hence, intensive activity does not predispose you to arthritis any more than intensive activity predisposes you to heart disease. Increasing evidence, based on careful studies of long-distance runners, who get very little arthritis, suggests that the very opposite may be true.

FEATURES

The bony knobs that form around the end joints of the fingers are called *Heberden's nodes* after the British doctor who first described them. In the middle joints of the fingers similar knobs can be found. Usually the bony enlargement occurs slowly over a period of years and is not even noticed by the patient. In most cases all of the fingers are involved more or less equally.

There is an interesting variation of osteoarthritis in which the bony swelling occurs over only three or four weeks in a single finger joint. The sudden swelling will cause redness and soreness until the process is complete, then hurting will stop altogether. Then the same process may occur in another joint, and then another. This syndrome is seen in women in their forties, earlier than the more usual form of osteoarthritis. These patients frequently have other family members with the same problem. This "familial" form of osteoarthrosis doesn't really seem very much worse than other osteoarthrosis over the long run.

Osteoarthrosis of the spine doesn't cause symptoms unless there is pressure on one of the nerves or irritation of some of the other structures of the back. The section in Part III on low back pain describes these problems. If someone tells you that you have arthritis in your spine, don't assume that the pain you feel is necessarily related to that arthritis. Most people with X-rays showing arthritis of the spine don't have any problem at all.

Osteoarthritis of the weight-bearing joints, particularly the hip and knee, develops slowly and often involves both sides of the body. Pain in the joint may remain fairly constant or may wax and wane for a period of years. In severe cases walking may be difficult or even impossible. Fluid may accumulate in the affected joint giving it a swollen appearance, or a knee may wobble a bit when weight is placed on it. In the knee, the osteoarthrosis will usually affect one half of the joint—inner or outer—more than the other; this may result in the leg becoming bowed or splayed outward and cause difficulty in walking.

Tests

X-rays are important in evaluating osteoarthritis, although both doctor and patient have to realize that X-ray findings are far more common than symptoms. The two major findings on the X-ray are narrowing of the joint space and the presence of bony spurs. In addition, X-rays can sometimes show the holes through which the nerves pass and indicate whether or not these holes are narrowed.

X-rays pass right through cartilage. Hence, in a normal joint the X-ray looks as though the two bones are separated by a space. In reality the apparent space is filled with cartilage. As the cartilage is frayed, the apparent joint space on the X-ray narrows until the two bones may be seen to touch each other. *Osteophytes*, or spurs, are little bony growths that appear alongside the places where the cartilage has degenerated. It is as though the body is trying to react to a cartilage problem by providing more surface area for the joint, so as to distribute the weight more evenly. At any rate, the bony growth provides a larger joint surface.

In contrast to X-rays, blood tests aren't very helpful in osteoarthritis. There's nothing wrong with the rest of the body, so all tests are normal.

PROGNOSIS

Prognosis is usually good for osteoarthritis. When one thinks of an aging process one tends to think of a progressive condition that gets worse and worse. This is not necessarily the case. Osteoarthritis may get worse for a time, then become stable for a long period. A joint that has lost its cartilage may not function well at first, but with use the bone may be molded and polished so that a smooth and more functional joint develops. Even in the worst cases osteoarthritis progresses slowly. You have lots of time to think about what kinds of treatment are likely to help. If a surgical decision is needed, you have ample time to consider whether you want an operation or not. Crippling from osteoarthritis is relatively rare, and most individuals with osteoarthritis remain essentially free of symptoms.

TREATMENT

Joints should be exercised through their full range of motion several times a day. If weight-bearing joints are involved, body weight should be kept under control. Obesity accelerates the rate of damage to the diseased joint, particularly if the knees are involved. The most helpful exercises seem to be swimming and walking—activities that are easy, can be gradually increased, and are smooth rather than jerky. Exercise should be regular and should not hurt much. If you start getting some osteoarthritis it is a signal, *not* to begin to tone down your life, but to develop a sensible, regular exercise program to strengthen the bones and ligaments surrounding the affected joints and to preserve mobility in joints that are developing spurs.

Drug therapy is used to control discomfort. Aspirin (p. 115) in moderate doses is frequently helpful. Recently acetaminophen (Tylenol, p. 133), which is the safest analgesic drug, has been found to be just as good for many people as the more toxic alternatives. Ibuprofen (p. 126) and other anti-inflammatory drugs (p. 112) are helpful for some people. I avoid codeine and strong pain pills because pain is a signal to the body that helps protect a diseased joint; it is important that this signal is received. The next section describes the kinds of arthritis that can follow when pain is suppressed too vigorously.

Some kinds of devices can help. A cane may be helpful; less commonly, crutches are needed. Occasionally special shoes or lifts on one side of the foot may be helpful.

Most physicians believe that symptomatic osteoarthritis may be prevented to a large extent by good health habits. If you are active, if you maintain a lean body weight, if you exercise your muscles and joints regularly so as to nourish cartilage, and if you let your common sense tell you when you've overdone it and something hurts, your joints should last a long time. Like exercise of the heart muscle, exercise of the muscles and joints provides reserves for the occasional strenuous activities we all encounter. Exercise builds strong tissues that last a long time.

Injection of osteoarthritic joints with corticosteroids (p. 135) is occasionally helpful, as is removal of some fluid from an involved joint. Unfortunately injections often don't help much, since there isn't much inflammation to be suppressed. Injections should not be frequently repeated because the injection of cortisone may damage the cartilage and the bone. Recently injections with hyaluronic acid (e.g., Synvisc) have been used to help lubricate the joint and appear to be helpful in some patients with knee osteoarthritis.

Surgery can be dramatically effective for patients with severe osteoarthritis of the weight-bearing joints. The total-hip-replacement operation (p. 165) is the most important operation yet devised for any form of arthritis. Essentially all patients are free of pain after the surgery and many walk normally and engage in normal activities. The total-knee-replacement (p. 165) is a more recent operation that already gives far better results than knee surgery available just a few years ago. Surgery is not urgent, and you and your doctor will want to decide the point at which the discomfort or the limitation on your walking has become sufficient to warrant the discomfort, the costs, and the small risk associated with the operation.

If your problem is osteoarthritis, proceed to Part II, page 103.

Joints Without Nerves (Neuropathic Joints)

Although this kind of arthritis is rare, I include it here to indicate the problems that can arise from the relief of pain and to illustrate the principal features of joint protection.

A joint without a nerve supply is spectacularly affected. Cartilage degenerates, bone fractures and distorts, and the joint becomes all but useless. This may take only a few months or a few years. Such joints are often called *Charcot joints,* after the physician who first described them in patients with syphilis.

What connection does this incredible arthritis have with the absence of a nerve supply to the joint? The answer is that normal activities impose tremendous stresses across our joints, but these forces are cushioned by nervous reflexes of which we are not even aware. If you were to jump from a stool two feet (60 cm) high and land on a hard surface with your knees locked, the stress across your knee joint would briefly reach several tons and you might be injured. On the other hand, your joints can tolerate a much higher jump quite readily if the fall is anticipated with bent knees and just the right amount of muscle tension at the time of impact. When we walk or climb stairs, the same thing happens in miniature. Potentially large stresses are absorbed by cushioning actions that require unconscious nervous reflexes. Tiny fibers in the joint and in the limbs tell the brain the position of the limb, and the brain then feeds back nerve impulses that prepare the joint for the next motion or impact. If these reflex nervous arcs are not present because of disease, the joint is quickly destroyed.

With syphilis affecting the nervous system, these reflex arcs may be interrupted. And with certain other diseases of the nervous system, the reflexes can be decreased. All of these conditions are rare, and you don't need to begin worrying about having any of them.

The importance of this discussion is in discovering the importance of pain. Pain is probably the body's single most important defense mechanism. It tells us when something is wrong. In the case of the joints, pain often tells us not to use a particular joint so much, to give it a rest for a while. The nerve fibers that tell the brain about position are not exactly the same as those that tell about pain, but they are closely related and they are affected by the same kinds of drugs. If you block these reflexes by using too many painkillers, you act to destroy your joints and to prevent your body from helping you minimize the damage. By causing more damage to the joint you cause more future pain for yourself, so that the drug giving you temporary pain relief may actually be increasing the amount of pain you will have during your life. Always think about the long-term effects of drug use, not just the immediate ones.

FEATURES

Charcot joints affect one or both knees, although other weight-bearing joints may be affected. The affected joint is massively swollen, distorted, and unstable. In the leg below the affected joint there is loss of nerve connections, and the physician can find a defect in pain and position perception. The X-rays show loss of cartilage, new bone growth, and frequently fractures at the joint. There are no laboratory test abnormalities in these conditions except those of the underlying disease that caused the nerve damage.

PROGNOSIS

This is a severe form of arthritis, and it usually will progress to serious disability, particularly at the knee. The prognosis is that of the disease that caused the nerve problem, such as syphilis or diabetes.

TREATMENT

The underlying disease may be treated effectively if it is syphilis and to some extent if it is diabetes. However, the nerves will not regenerate after treatment of the disease and the joint problem may continue to get worse.

Protection of the joints with crutches or a cane and limited use of the joints are important. Drugs do not help much. Surgery is only rarely attempted and only moderately successful. Artificial joints won't work very well here because of the pounding they take, but fusion of the joint can sometimes help.

If your problem is neuropathic joints, proceed to Part II, page 103.

CHAPTER 8

Muscle Inflammation

Inflammation in the Muscle Fibers

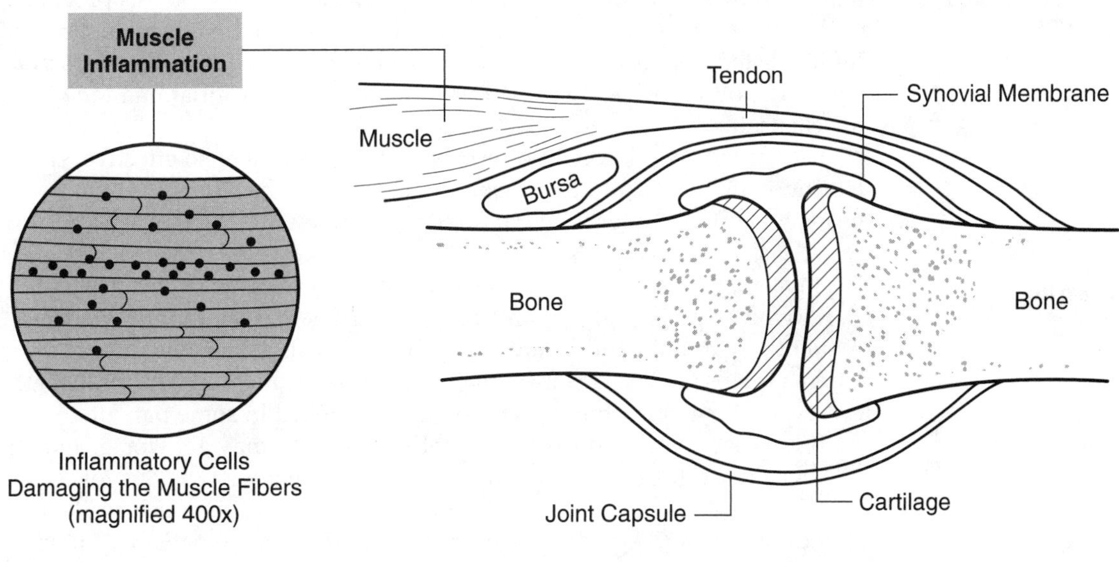

Inflammatory Cells Damaging the Muscle Fibers (magnified 400x)

Near the joint, the muscles may become inflamed. Here, in **polymyositis (PM)** or **dermatomyositis (DM),** the inflammatory cells may be seen between and injuring the muscle fibers. In **polymyalgia rheumatica (PMR)** the muscles are again involved, but the inflammation is in the small blood vessels and is harder to see under the microscope.

Polymyalgia Rheumatica (PMR)

When an older person develops severe aching of the muscles, it may be *polymyalgia rheumatica.* This is a fairly common kind of rheumatism. It is a serious condition but the treatment for it is extremely effective. Hence, it is important to know a little bit about it.

Let's take a look at those long words. The prefix *poly* means "many." The root *my* in the middle of the word means "muscle." The ending *algia* denotes "pain." So the first long word means "pain in many muscles." The second word, *rheumatica,* just tells us redundantly that the aching and pain are those we often associate with the rather vague term *rheumatism.*

This syndrome was recognized in the United States in the late 1960s. The cause is unknown, but the pain and disability seem related to inflammation of the small blood vessels that supply the muscles. So it is probably an *arteritis*—that is, an arterial inflammation—rather than a muscle disease. But it is listed here because the muscle aching is the major feature. It is not related to polymyositis, discussed next, which involves inflammation of the muscle itself.

Because the condition is so serious and the treatment so effective, early detection, diagnosis, and treatment are important. The disease is by no means rare. One in every several hundred people will experience it.

FEATURES

Polymyalgia rheumatica causes muscle aching in persons over the age of 50. It involves principally the muscles of the neck and shoulder regions, frequently with pain and aching in the hip areas also. The average age of patients is close to 70. The onset may be gradual or may occur over just a few days. Morning stiffness **(S2)** can be pronounced in some patients.

If not diagnosed and treated early the condition may get worse, and may even resemble cancer. Patients may be tired, have low fevers for a long time, and lose significant amounts of weight, even as much as 30 or 40 pounds (14 to 18 kg). There can be a synovitis in some patients, so the joints as well as the muscles ache.

The artery inflammation found in some patients may affect the arteries of the temples. There may be pain or visible redness over these arteries, and they may hurt when pressed. Using the affected muscles, as in using the arm repeatedly or in chewing a thick steak, may cause pain due to inadequacy of blood supply. In rare cases the artery to the eye can be affected, causing blindness in the eye. This is the most serious complication of the disease. When artery inflammation is found this disease is potentially more severe and is called *giant-cell arteritis.*

Tests

In the laboratory, the sedimentation rate is greatly elevated. Indeed, this test is higher in polymyalgia rheumatica than in any other disease. Additionally, the level of *fibrinogen*, a soluble protein in the blood, may be raised, and the patient is often anemic, sometimes severely.

Biopsies of the arteries are sometimes helpful for diagnosis, but biopsy of the muscle shows surprisingly little damage under the microscope. A biopsy of the temporal artery can sometimes prove the diagnosis of giant-cell arteritis.

There are no X-ray changes characteristic of polymyalgia rheumatica.

PROGNOSIS

Without treatment this condition appears to last three to five years on the average, gradually disappearing thereafter. During that period all patients will have been very symptomatic and a few will have lost vision in one or both eyes.

With treatment, on the other hand, the patient is immediately nearly well, typically within two days of beginning treatment. Blindness after treatment is exceedingly rare, and complications from treatment are relatively unusual.

Polymyalgia can be very similar to rheumatoid arthritis that starts in the later years. Some patients will be found after several months or years to have actually had rheumatoid arthritis.

TREATMENT

The cornerstone of treatment is corticosteroid medication. The drug usually chosen is prednisone (p. 137), and it is started at a medium or high dosage depending on the severity of the case. It is then rapidly decreased to lower doses, which must be maintained for some time. Prednisone is typically required for eighteen months to three years, occasionally longer. The prednisone does not cure the disease but is successful in entirely eliminating the symptoms.

Usually the increase in activity afforded by the prednisone is so substantial that it makes up for any side effects that might occur. There does seem to be a slight tendency for patients on prednisone to develop the shingles. Some patients may suffer some osteoporosis or softening of the bones and may have fractures, particularly of the spine.

The response to treatment is absolutely dramatic. Polymyalgia rheumatica frequently affects individuals who have been active throughout their lives, leaving them very disturbed by their inability to engage in their favorite activities. A patient who loves to play golf, for example, and has been unable to play for the past six months because of pain in the shoulders and neck is likely to become depressed and discouraged. Usually patients will suggest that it must be "old age" catching up with them. But such patients may be back on the golf course the day after therapy is begun.

Because the response to prednisone is so very striking, some physicians have suggested using less dangerous anti-inflammatory agents such as aspirin (p. 115) or indomethacin (p. 124) for milder cases of polymyalgia rheumatica. In a few instances such treatment has been successful, but most doctors prefer to treat this condition definitively with prednisone. Other drugs, such as methotrexate, are occasionally used.

No restrictions on activity are required, and patients may resume their normal activities after treatment. As the corticosteroid is decreased and eventually discontinued, it is not unusual for some mild symptoms to return, but these usually pose little problem. The most bothersome side effect of the prednisone is loss of calcium from the bones, causing osteoporosis. For this reason many physicians like to prescribe calcium supplements and vitamin D to attempt to prevent this complication. Weight-bearing activity, such as walking, is also very important in fighting osteoporosis.

If your problem is polymyalgia rheumatica, proceed to Part II, page 103.

Polymyositis (PM) and Dermatomyositis (DM)

Polymyositis and its close relative *dermatomyositis* are diseases of the muscle and skin that cause not only pain but also weakness and destruction of the muscle. The inflammation (*itis*) in the muscles results in destruction of the muscle fibers.

Along with this process in the muscles most patients have some involvement of the skin, with skin rash and changes in the skin blood vessels. While the cause of polymyositis is not known, the damage appears to occur because the body's blood cell lymphocytes have become sensitized to the person's own muscle and attack that muscle.

FEATURES

These muscle disorders can occur in any age group and in either sex. In childhood dermatomyositis, the muscle weakness is profound and, after years, the damaged muscles may be permanently replaced by calcium deposits (*calcinoses*) that can further limit motion.

Because this is predominately a disease of muscles, weakness is the biggest problem. It affects many muscles throughout the body, particularly those of the upper arms, upper legs, and neck region. The involved muscles are weak, frequently tender, and frequently painful. The weakness is often such that the patient cannot get up from a straight chair without assistance and may not be able to lift the head from the bed while lying flat. Problems with the upper swallowing muscles can cause a nasal speech pattern and difficulty in swallowing solid foods. Patients may have trouble climbing stairs or holding their arms out straight to the side.

The skin can be involved. The blood vessels dilate, giving an unusual lavender or heliotrope color to the skin in certain areas. Most frequently these areas are the eyelids, the knuckles, and the ends of the fingers around the fingernails. A red rash may occur over much of the rest of the body. There may be some swelling in these regions, but the color changes are most characteristic. Other body organs can be involved; most troublesome is involvement of the lungs. The fingers may be afflicted with Raynaud's phenomenon, in which they turn white and blue in response to cold.

Although the lungs are not often directly involved they nevertheless constitute the major problem. Weakness in the swallowing muscles or in the breathing muscles can lead to swallowing food "the wrong way," into the lungs, or the inability to breathe energetically enough.

Dermatomyositis and polymyositis can be caused by underlying cancer, although this is quite unusual. It is extremely rare to find a tumor in a patient below the age of 50, and only 10 to 20% of cases over that age are associated with tumors.

Tests

In the laboratory the main clues to the disease are found by tests of muscle enzymes. Two enzymes in particular, creatine phosphokinase (CPK) and aldolase, are usually elevated. (Other enzymes that may be elevated include the SGOT and SGPT.) Other tests are less rewarding: The sedimentation rate may be elevated or not, the blood counts are usually normal, and abnormal antibodies or rheumatoid factors are usually absent. X-rays help very little since the soft tissues do not show up well on X-ray. An exception is the chest X-ray, which can provide some information about involvement of the lungs. Calcinosis can also be seen on X-ray. Another test, the electromyogram, tests the electrical function of the nerves and muscles. Sometimes this test will help to distinguish polymyositis from a disease of the nerves.

Biopsy of the muscle, in which a small piece of a leg muscle or an upper arm muscle is inspected under the microscope, is the definitive test. Inflammation in the muscle is vividly seen under the microscope. Unfortunately, since the disease does not affect every muscle equally, a negative biopsy may indicate merely that a diseased spot was missed. If a weak and tender muscle is biopsied, the result will usually be positive.

PROGNOSIS

This is a serious but variably severe disease. It is a connective-tissue disease and, as such, is more than just arthritis or rheumatism. In fact, many people would not call it a form of arthritis at all since the joints are not often involved. Some patients die within five years of the start of the disease; this mortality includes many older patients who have a cancer associated with their disease. On the other hand, many other patients do extremely well. They may respond quickly to treatment, the disease may go away, and, after a period of months, the medicine may be discontinued and they may return to totally normal living. Such cases of polymyositis are "one-shot"—a single episode of illness that lasts some months, then disappears, never to recur. Other patients have a progressive form that can be difficult to treat.

The greatest dangers of polymyositis come from involvement of the lungs. Because the muscles in the chest wall are weak, breathing is weak and the patient may not be able to get enough oxygen. Further, since the swallowing mechanism in the throat can be weakened, food may accidentally be inhaled into the lungs and cause a serious pneumonia. So patients without involvement of the lungs or of the swallowing muscles have a better prognosis.

TREATMENT

The mainstay of treatment used to be corticosteroid medication, usually prednisone (p. 137). These powerful drugs are given to almost all patients and usually result in return of the muscle enzymes to normal over several weeks and a gradual increase in muscle strength over the following two to twelve months. Usually the steroids are then tapered to lower doses to decrease toxic reactions. Unfortunately, when steroids are used for long periods in high doses they cause wasting and weakness of the muscles. There is potential danger that the medicine may contribute to weakness in a disease that already has weakness as its principal problem. Aspirin (p. 115) and other anti-inflammatory drugs are occasionally used to reduce muscle inflammation.

If the disease is not easily controlled with prednisone or if the prednisone cannot be tapered to less toxic levels, most physicians will add immunosuppressant drugs. These are frequently successful. Most commonly used is methotrexate (p. 150), and this has become the most useful drug for myositis. Azathioprine (Imuran, p. 151) is another frequently used immunosuppressant agent. There is an increasing tendency to rely on these drugs (particularly methotrexate) instead of prednisone because they are often more effective and less toxic.

There is controversy about how long patients require treatment. Some physicians feel that most patients need to continue treatment for life. In our clinic, approximately half of our patients get off medication within several years. A patient with this disease, however, should expect to be taking medication for some time.

Exercise

There has also been controversy about the role of exercise in polymyositis. It has been pointed out that exercise will increase the inflammation slightly and will increase the blood levels of the muscle enzymes, which are already abnormally high. On the other hand, exercise preserves the function of the muscles and provides a stimulus to make the muscles stronger. We tell our patients to exercise regularly but gently, gradually increasing the scope of their activities. All of the affected muscles should be worked through their entire range of motion each day to prevent stiffness. Steady exercise to build up strength can consist of walking or swimming or bicycling. We prefer that patients don't overdo exercise until they are conditioned but that they build slowly toward a stronger exercise program with the goal of restoring normal strength.

It is crucial for the patient to recognize that the process of regaining strength is a very long one. Any time the muscle system is out of condition the retraining process is lengthy. The body must put many pounds of muscle together, and that muscle must become trained and mature. Even without a disease it may take six to twelve months to regain strength after an enforced period of idleness; with myositis this period may be even longer. The patient should continue to increase activity but should not expect that return of full strength or of a normal muscular appearance will occur over a short period.

Smoking, because it injures the lungs, should be discontinued. Patients with Raynaud's phenomenon should keep generally warm and take care of their hands, which will be sensitive to damage from the cold. Patients with trouble swallowing who run the risk of aspiration pneumonia should eat their meals sitting up. They should remain in a sitting or standing position until two or three hours after the last meal of the day, so the stomach has a chance to empty before they lie down. Eating softer foods that pass more easily through the digestive tract may also be helpful.

If your problem is polymyositis or dermatomyositis, proceed to Part II, page 103.

CHAPTER 9

Local Conditions
Injury, Inflammation, and Repair

Detailed discussion of certain local conditions and their treatment, other than those featured in this chapter, appears in Part III. The following list suggests some of these problems.

- Metatarsalgia (ball of the foot)—page 212
- Achilles tendinitis (heel)—page 214
- Heel-spur syndrome—page 214
- Sprained ankle—page 216
- Cervical neck strain—page 224
- Frozen shoulder—page 227
- Tennis elbow—page 230
- Carpal tunnel syndrome (wrist)—page 232

Bursitis

A *bursa* is a small sac of tissue similar to the synovial tissue that lines the joints. The bursa sac contains a lubricating fluid, and the bursa is designed to ease the movement of muscle across muscle or of muscle across bone. A bursa does not connect to the joint space of a nearby joint but is a separate sac. Bursae can become inflamed as part of a general inflammation of the synovial tissue, but usually an individual experiences bursitis in one or two bursae at a time rather than as part of a major disease process.

"Housemaid's knee" is an outdated term for *prepatellar bursitis,* in which the bursa in front of and just below the kneecap is inflamed. *Olecranon bursitis* occurs over the point of the elbow, and sometimes a fluid-filled sac may be visible at that point. *Subdeltoid bursitis* occurs in the shoulder—or more precisely, the outer aspect of the upper arm. There are literally dozens of similar bursae in the body, and any of them can become inflamed in a particular instance.

FEATURES

Bursitis is an inflammation of a bursa and results in localized pain. Sometimes the pain is on both sides of the body, as with both knees. There is pain when the inflamed area is pressed, and heat or redness is common. If the bursa is located close enough to the skin, swelling can be seen.

Bursitis comes on relatively suddenly, within hours to days. It frequently follows injury to the area, repeated pressure on the area, or overuse. In the shoulder particularly it may be associated with tendinitis or calcific tendinitis, and can be part of the "frozen shoulder" problem (see Shoulder Pain, **S14**).

PROGNOSIS

Almost all episodes of bursitis will subside within several days to several weeks, but they may recur. If the process causing the bursitis is continued the bursitis may persist; otherwise, it follows a normal healing course over a period of one week to ten days. Some people seem more prone to bursitis than others and have recurrent problems throughout their lives. If the affected part is held rigid, some residual stiffness may result; otherwise, no crippling whatsoever should result from bursitis.

TREATMENT

If the problem is tolerable, treat it with "tincture of time." Wait for the body to control and heal the process. Avoid the precipitating cause if you are able to identify it. Use drugs very sparingly; the process is local, and systemic drugs like aspirin are not very helpful. Resting the part will speed reduction of the inflammation, and you may want to use a sling or other device to increase the rest. Gentle warmth provided by a heating pad or warm bath frequently makes the bursitis feel better. The affected area should be worked through its full range of motion several times daily, even if it is a bit tender, to prevent stiffness developing in the part. But remember, patience and avoidance of reinjury are the major tactics.

If the discomfort persists for a number of weeks despite the measures outlined above, see the doctor. The doctor may recommend that you continue the same general measures discussed here. Alternatively an anti-inflammatory agent may be prescribed; these help a few people but are generally just a way of buying a little more patience from the patient. Finally, the doctor may inject the bursa with corticosteroids (p. 135). These injections are usually successful and not overly painful. They are relatively free of side effects and most physicians feel they are appropriate treatment for a local condition if it is severe and has persisted.

For a local problem as above, read about the particular problem in Part III.

Low Back Syndromes

Pain in the low back has been called the "curse of the erect posture." From an engineering standpoint, when humans developed a standing posture the spine developed a double bend, concave in the lower back and convex in the upper back. The back is a complex mechanism with hundreds of ligaments and scores of joints; it should not be surprising that injury to this complicated organ occurs in over one-half of all people. Pain can be extremely severe and has been compared with the pain of childbirth, kidney stones, or a heart attack. Low back pain results in as much long-term disability and as many days lost from work as does almost any other illness or injury. Yet as we will see, it is always difficult to be sure what is going on in an individual case. Further discussion of back pain can be found in Low Back Pain, **S12.**

The spine consists of a stack of bones, the *vertebrae.* Disks separate individual vertebrae much like mushrooms between pieces of steak on a shish kebab. Each vertebra is connected to the next one by ligaments that cross the vertebral disks. Long ligaments run up and down the length of the spine. Muscles and shoulder ligaments attach each vertebra to the ones directly adjacent; other muscles and ligaments bridge two vertebrae, and three, and four, and so forth. In addition to the disks separating the vertebrae, there are small joints that provide two additional points of contact and movement. These small joints are bridged by ligaments and have synovial tissue within them just like larger joints.

Most low back syndromes are due to problems with one of the back parts mentioned above—the ligaments, the muscles, the joint synovium, or the joint ligaments. (Problems with the disk itself will be discussed in the following section.) Additionally, obese people may have little ruptures of fat through the back tissues, and these may cause pain.

All minor injuries of the back look and act about the same. A major disk problem, a *herniated nucleus pulposis,* is different and may involve nerve injury. From the outside, neither the doctor nor the patient can tell exactly which tissue was initially injured. Wherever the problem started, a larger portion of the back becomes involved as the body works to immobilize the part to allow its healing. In such cases, muscle spasm and widespread pain are the rule.

FEATURES

Low back syndromes usually result from an injury. The injury is usually obvious, but in at least one-third of patients no incident can be remembered. Muscle spasm provides protection for the injured part by helping to immobilize the back, but this spasm is itself painful. Except for the spasm, which is unique to the back, think of a low back problem as analogous to the more familiar sprain of an ankle. The pain and local swelling are maximum within 24 hours, remain acute and severe for 24 to 72 hours, are somewhat nagging for another week, and require perhaps 6 weeks to heal back to full strength. Reinjury is very common and starts the timetable all over again. Frequent reinjury can lead to chronic sprains that are more difficult to treat and take a longer time to heal.

The pain is usually most pronounced in the concave portion of the lower back and may frequently radiate to the buttocks. There is pain in the areas of muscle spasm, and on subsequent days, the pain may rise higher in the back as the tired muscles that have been in spasm begin to complain loudly. The pain should not go down into the calf; if it does run down a leg, it is a reason to see the doctor.

The most frequent injury is a sudden hyperextension, in which the lower body continues forward and the upper body is suddenly arched backward. However, all kinds of injuries can result in these syndromes. Injuries occur most frequently in the overweight or inactive individual, or in the individual who exercises only episodically. Good muscle tone and regular exercise protect the back and decrease the risk of these conditions.

PROGNOSIS

About half of patients with low back syndromes have only one to three episodes over a lifetime; the remainder have more episodes than this. Prognosis for the individual episode is excellent, and the chances of a serious problem involving pressure on nerves or requiring spinal surgery are less than 1%. If the pain runs down into the legs, particularly the outside of the legs and particularly below the knee, the prognosis is more guarded, and greater care in management and in the consideration of surgery is necessary.

If the pain is somewhat less dramatic but lasts for a period of many weeks or months, is worst in the morning, is rather slow in developing, gets better with exercise during the day, and occurs in a person below age 40, ankylosing spondylitis, (pp. 35–39) should be suspected. Common low back syndromes may loosen up a little bit with activity but by and large get worse if you overdo before the healing is complete.

TREATMENT

The primary goal in treating an acute low back problem is to prevent a chronic low back problem. The injury must heal and this takes time. For the acute painful problem, two possible treatment strategies are acceptable. A third one is not. First, there is the "least pain" strategy. This involves bed rest, a bed board to provide firm support, sometimes a small pillow beneath the low back if this increases comfort, heat beginning the second day, and pain relievers and muscle relaxants as required to increase comfort.

The second is the "natural" strategy, in which the patient is up and around as the pain allows, avoids pain relievers, and does not use muscle relaxants. If you can stand the often severe pain, this way may be best.

The third (and unacceptable) strategy is "reinjury," in which the patient is up and around and also uses pain relievers and muscle relaxants. The body will heal low back syndrome if left alone. However, if you blunt the pain response of the body and interfere with the immobilization provided naturally by muscle spasm, then reinjury is likely and will delay healing.

You can prevent reinjury by greatly limiting activity—this is the "least pain" way. Or you can prevent reinjury by allowing the pain reflex and the muscle spasm to protect the injured point—this is the "natural" way. But if you combine these strategies, you are asking for a long-term problem.

After the acute injury is over, it is time to begin thinking about preventing the next one. Control of weight involves not only reducing to a good body weight but also constant maintenance of that weight. Development of gentle, regular, graded activity to strengthen the spine and improve muscle tone is important. Back protection techniques can help prevent injury when lifting or using the back for different tasks. And specific back exercises can help to strengthen the muscles on the outside of the back and also those that are inside and unseen. By gradually increasing activity, most patients with low back syndromes can return to any activity desired. Even horseback riding and heavy labor are entirely possible if the progression to full activity is patient and gradual. Low Back Pain, **S12,** discusses these treatment approaches in greater detail.

Herniated Lumbar Disk

Aye, there's the rub. The problem with herniated disks is that they can rub on nerves and cause nerve damage, with serious problems down the leg in areas distant from the back. Luckily, few back problems are actually herniated lumbar disks, and most herniated disks will get better without surgery. Many physicians think that lumbar disks are overdiagnosed and perhaps overtreated. The potential problem is the compression of the nerves, and the following discussion should help you understand this problem.

The stack of vertebrae in the spine are separated by fibrous intervertebral disks, each about one-third inch (0.8 cm) in height. The outer portion of this disk is fibrous tissue called the *annulus fibrosis,* and the center portion is a softer, more gelatinous material called the *nucleus pulposis.* This forms an energy-absorbing yet flexible material that helps cushion the spine while allowing it to move in a supple fashion. Above and below the intervertebral disks are the cartilage end plates of the vertebrae; these are thin layers of cartilage that surface the bones. With increasing age and increasing cumulative injury to the spine, the disk becomes a bit more scarred in the center and a bit narrower. Osteoarthrosis changes can occur next to the disk, with bone spurs growing out from the vertebrae. This process is very slow and usually doesn't cause any symptoms. It does make us get about an inch (2.5 cm) shorter as we grow older.

A major problem occurs when the gelatinous material in the center of the disk pushes out, or herniates, through a tear in weakened fibers. This is a little bit like what happens with the filling when you bite into a chocolate eclair. When there is a sudden herniation of the disk, a glob of the interior disk substance is now on the outside of the disk.

This glob would eventually be reabsorbed by normal body mechanisms without symptoms, leaving a slightly narrower disk space. But the herniated disk material can press on the nerves that go out from the spine, and that's where the rub comes in.

FEATURES

Acute herniated disks tend to occur in the third or fourth decade of life and less frequently in older individuals. In later life a disk that is degenerated has become scarred and cannot rupture any longer.

A disk can rupture at any level of the spine, but most frequently one of the bottom two disks is involved. These are the disk between the sacrum and the lowest lumbar vertebra and the disk between the fourth and fifth lumbar vertebrae, both in the low back. Usually the rupture will occur just to one side of the midline in the back part of the disk. This is an area that is relatively undefended by other ligaments. It can happen on either side, but usually not on both sides at once.

Very rarely, the disk will rupture in the middle and cause immediate severe nerve problems by compressing all of the contents of the spinal canal. Patients with this condition suffer back pain as well as an immediate inability to urinate; in this situation (and this situation alone) immediate surgery is required.

The more classical kind of nerve compression affects just one side and results in *sciatica,* which is irritation of some of the fibers that lead to the sciatic nerve. Depending on how much compression and at what level of the spine the injury occurred, there may be loss of the reflexes in the leg, numbness of the leg, paralysis or weakness of parts, or total loss of feeling in some areas. Pain is frequently aggravated by a cough or a sneeze, and raising the straightened leg on the affected side increases the pain, often dramatically.

Many patients describe two different kinds of pain. One is a deep, aching pain in the back that runs down the back of the affected buttock. The other is a sharp, needlelike pain that runs down the outside of the leg, beyond the knee, down the outer part of the calf, and into the outer portion of the foot.

The back is frequently in spasm as it is with any back injury, and it will assume a position (curvature of the spine) that relieves the pressure on the nerve root. Thus, the spasm can help prevent nerve damage.

Some doctors feel that a number of the minor back problems discussed in the previous section are actually disk protrusions that do not cause nerve pressure. This may well be true, but there is no reason to consider a disk problem more serious than these other problems unless some symptoms of rubbing on the nerve roots are present. Nor should expensive major diagnostic tests such as magnetic resonance (MR) imaging be required in routine cases.

PROGNOSIS

Surgery is recommended for between 5% and 30% of patients with nerve root compression, this figure depending partly on the particular doctor consulted. We feel that the lower figures are more appropriate and that back surgery should be carefully considered and reconsidered, preferably with two or more physicians' opinions, before the final surgical decision is made. It is well known that the back problem may recur even after surgery, if not at the disk that was removed then at another level. Further, the back surgery itself disrupts at least a part of this very complex body part and can result in some scarring and stiffness.

Most people with disk problems recover without surgery, and most are able to return to work and eventually to full activity. The time required may be discouragingly long—many weeks or months—but the motivated and careful patient will usually achieve good results without surgery.

TREATMENT

Bed rest, in the position of greatest comfort, is central to most treatment. Some doctors recommend a pillow under the knees or under the low back; others emphasize a straight, firm bed board. The key is the position of greatest comfort. Pain medications may be required, but as emphasized in the previous section, they should not be used to allow activity that would otherwise not be possible since this may encourage more nerve damage and slower healing.

Manipulation is employed by some doctors and other practitioners. Several maneuvers are used, including straight leg raising on the affected side, bending the knees back to the chest and pushing on them with a circular motion, and backward stretching. These procedures sometimes work—with a little pop, the symptoms go away. Presumably what happens is that the herniated material shifts position slightly, relieving the pressure on the nerve. Unfortunately the potential exists for completely breaking the nerve root by these maneuvers, and we recommend that they be undertaken only by an experienced professional. All patients with symptoms of nerve root compression should be under a doctor's care.

Hospital bed rest may be required in a few cases. Some physicians use traction but others argue strongly against it. Some physicians employ a corset to help support the spine; we have not had a great deal of success with corsets.

Surgery is required for patients with urine retention or major nerve syndromes. The surgery is usually successful in relieving the immediate nerve pressure, but problems can recur and back pain may persist.

In the asymptomatic interval following healing of an acute disk injury, exercises to strengthen the paraspinal muscles are helpful, and carefully graded return to activity is important.

If you have a back problem, check any drugs required in chapters 14, 15, and 16, then proceed to Part III.

CHAPTER 10

General Conditions
Aching and Tender All Over

A whole host of disease conditions have been termed *nonarticular rheumatism,* a most unfortunate and confusing term. It means "rheumatism not involving the joints." The various terms—*fibromyalgia, psychogenic rheumatism, psycho-physiological musculoskeletal reaction, anxiety neurosis, depressive reaction*—are just as confusing. None of these terms is particularly accurate, and none of them can be applied to all patients with symptoms of long-term general aching and the total absence of evidence of an actual disease process. The patient is confused by these conditions—in part because the doctor is likely to be confused. There are no really clear distinctions in this disease area.

The discussion in this chapter falls under three headings: fibromyalgia, psychogenic rheumatism, and depression and arthritis. These distinctions are not always clear, and you may want to read each section carefully to see which aspects of the discussion seem to apply to you.

Part of the frustration of these syndromes is that they are "nonobjective"; that is, with the exception of tender points, nothing in the physical examination or in the laboratory examination suggests that anything at all is wrong with the patient. Further, nothing really happens to the patient as time goes on. The frustrating symptoms may go away or stay, but they don't get worse. Over time most of the symptoms eventually disappear. Research has given us some insights into the condition originally called fibrositis but now known as fibromyalgia; this condition now has the characteristics of an understandable disease. Nevertheless, none of the theories about the conditions discussed below is totally convincing.

Fibromyalgia

Fibromyalgia is a common and increasingly recognized condition. In 1990 it was defined in terms of two distinguishing characteristics:

- Aching in many parts of the body lasting for at least 3 months
- Tenderness in 11 of 18 specified places on the body

FEATURES

The fibromyalgia syndrome (FMS) affects perhaps 5 million people in the United States and accounts for one out of every six visits to rheumatologists. Patients are more likely to be women, but children, the elderly, and men can also be affected. Their average age is about 55. People with this syndrome also may experience sleep disturbances, severe fatigue, morning stiffness, irritable bowel syndrome, anxiety, and other symptoms, such as trouble remembering things.

Many readers will be able to identify the *tender points* on their own bodies. Firm pressure applied to them will hurt anyone, but the person with fibromyalgia experiences great pain when these areas are pressed lightly. For example, about halfway between the neck and the shoulder, one can feel the upper border of the trapezius muscle; at the midpoint of this muscle there is a tender site. The "tennis elbow" site is about an inch (2.5 cm) down the forearm from the outer bump on the side of the elbow when the palm is turned up; this tender spot may feel like a cord. There is also tenderness next to either side of the breastbone and about an inch or two (2 to 5 cm) below the collarbone. A fourth site is in the fat pad inside the knee. Others are between the shoulder blades and at the base of the skull. A person with fibromyalgia usually has tenderness at most of these places and may have widespread tenderness as well.

Half or more of those with fibromyalgia have chronic fatigue. Fatigue may be severe and interfere with activities. Pain, sleep problems, and stress factors contribute to fatigue. A frequent but not quite universal characteristic of fibromyalgia is sleep disturbance. There is an interruption of slow-wave brain activity, the kind of sleep most restful to the muscles, in many patients. Upon awakening, patients may feel as though they never got to sleep at all.

Although the cause of fibromyalgia is unknown, researchers have several theories. It may be that there is a new "thermostat" setting for the pain threshold in fibromyalgia patients, who have more of a particular pain peptide (substance P) in their cerebrospinal fluid. Serotonin in the platelets is lower than normal. Some believe fibromyalgia may be associated with changes in muscle metabolism such as decreased blood flow, causing fatigue and decreased strength. Others believe that the syndrome may be triggered by an infectious agent, such as a virus. Stress is also frequently reported as a cause.

We recommend an excellent book, *The Fibromyalgia Help Book,* by Jenny Fransen and I. John Russell (St. Paul, Minn.: Smith House Press, 1996). A good video is available through Fibromyalgia Information Resources, P.O. Box 690402, San Antonio, TX 78269.

PROGNOSIS

Medically, fibromyalgia carries a fairly good prognosis for most people. There will usually be no crippling, but the discomfort may last for many years or even for life. The pain can vary over months or years but often never fully goes away. Most fibromyalgia patients are able to work. About 30% have had to reduce the duration or physical exertion associated with their jobs. About 15% are disabled and receiving Social Security disability payments.

Fibromyalgia symptoms may also be seen in many other disease conditions, such as rheumatoid arthritis or lupus, which themselves may disturb sleep. This "secondary" fibromyalgia must not be confused with a flare-up of the other condition, since the treatment is different.

TREATMENT

Treatment for fibromyalgia is usually frustrating for both the patient and the doctor. Often the patient's close family are equally frustrated. The root cause of the frustration is the difficulty in getting the symptoms to go away.

The doctor is frustrated for many reasons. There are no objective findings to observe. All the trusted tests are negative. Familiar treatments such as anti-inflammatory medications and analgesics don't work well. The doctor may not even believe that the condition fibromyalgia exists. The patient is often angry and demanding. When therapy is suggested, the patient often tells the doctor that it won't work, even before it has been tried. The doctor finds it all too easy to conclude that "it's all in your head."

The person with fibromyalgia is even more frustrated. She or he hurts. The job, the family, the satisfactions of life are threatened. Drug after drug fails to help. Exercise seems to cause flare-ups. The doctor doesn't get it. The doctor doesn't listen. The patient has trouble being taken seriously. The doctor thinks "it's all in your head" while the patient desperately wants the problem taken care of.

Fibromyalgia is a real condition, and the symptoms are real, chronic, and frustrating. They are *not* "all in your head." Chronic pain does affect your mental and emotional state, and frustration and anger do not help. You need a doctor who listens, cares, and communicates. The doctor needs a patient who works persistently at the self-management program. There is no magic, but there is help.

Exercise, slowly increased toward full aerobic conditioning and physical tiredness, is the most important component of treatment (see Chapter 13). Start slowly—even a minute or two an hour is helpful if you have been completely inactive. When a patient can walk extensively and swim, hike, or bicycle regularly, we sometimes see gradual resolution of the problem in only a few months. In general, impact exercises such as jogging, tennis, or basketball should be avoided. Stretching exercises are important. Pain often gets worse before it gets better with a new exercise program. Studies have shown that aerobic exercise improves muscle fitness and reduces muscle pain and tenderness. It may also improve sleep.

Progressive muscle relaxation or some other structured relaxation program may also be helpful. Heat and massage may give short-term relief. Pain management programs may be beneficial; the most success has come from psychological interventions that include cognitive behavioral therapy. Check with your local chapter of The Arthritis Foundation or The Arthritis Society for information about fibromyalgia support groups.

Medications that have proved most effective are generally given an hour before bedtime and include amitriptyline (Elavil), cyclobenzaprine (Flexeril), alprazolam (Xanax), and Soma. While these drugs have anti-depressive properties, they are not given for depression but to improve sleep quality and to relax muscles. These medications increase deep sleep. Ordinary "sleeping pills" are generally not helpful. Nonsteroidal drugs such as ibuprofen or naproxen are often used, with variable success. An increasingly common regimen is Prozac in the morning and Elavil in the evening. Side effects of medications are common but can often be avoided with lower doses and a different schedule. Some authorities recommend vitamin B_1 and B_6 supplements, and benefit has been reported with a combination of magnesium and malic acid.

Psychogenic Rheumatism

The pain fibers linking the body to the brain are continually firing off impulses about some sensation or another. Usually we suppress and ignore these signals if they are too minor to merit attention. But if we sit quietly and scan our bodies carefully for any painful signals, we can find some at any given moment.

Some people complain of "aching all over." On closer examination, it appears that while their painful sensations are not abnormal, their reaction to these sensations is. These normal sensations have become a medical problem. This is one explanation for psychogenic rheumatism, a very inadequately defined condition.

A frequent common denominator to these painful syndromes is accident litigation, disability insurance application, or the use of a painful symptom to manipulate another individual. This common denominator is called *secondary gain.* Pain, a normally undesirable symptom, assumes value because it helps in getting someone else to do what the individual wants. There is an incentive to amplify and pay attention to—rather than ignore—our normal minor pain impulses. The patient is very seldom aware that this is happening; this sequence is seldom a deliberate deception.

FEATURES

These syndromes can take several forms. The pain can be all over the body or in the area of a previous injury, often the neck (whiplash) or low back. Often patients report pains that do not follow anatomic patterns—that is, they don't follow the course of actual nerves.

Patients are often tense, sometimes angry. The syndrome may merge with fibromyalgia and the chronic fatigue syndrome.

Laboratory tests and X-rays are normal or, if abnormal, do not explain the symptoms. The symptoms do not respond well to medications or injections.

PROGNOSIS

Serious musculoskeletal problems are not possible, since this really is not a disease of the musculoskeletal system. The syndrome can be an unhappy one, however, and may persist for months or years. Drug dependency can result, and problems with excessive drug use or excessive surgery are the most unfortunate results.

TREATMENT

Crippling or major disability will not commonly result. Sometimes laboratory tests are ordered by the doctor in an effort to reassure the patient. It is important to honestly identify and to remove any secondary gain considerations. This syndrome notoriously improves as soon as a lawsuit is settled, whatever the outcome. It may respond to better, more direct communication between a manipulated person and the manipulator. Finally, avoidance of drugs is central to good therapy. Medication is not helpful and offers potential for dependency. Further, the mood-altering effects of commonly prescribed drugs make coping with this frustrating syndrome more difficult.

Depression and Arthritis

While we all get depressed sometimes, serious psychiatric depressions constitute major illness. The patient feels helpless and worthless. Everything is down, down, down. Sleep may be disturbed by obsessive, recurring, pessimistic thoughts. Speech and body movements are slow, and much of the body is frequently stiff. These pains and stiffness may be called "rheumatism" or "arthritis"; they are most frequent in older individuals.

Depressive reactions may follow loss of a loved one. These grief reactions, while similar to other depression, are ultimately less serious since they normally resolve after several months of adjustment.

FEATURES

This syndrome is a vague one. It may blend with psychogenic rheumatism or with fibromyalgia. The sleep deprivation mechanism that operates in fibromyalgia probably accentuates the symptoms. And the patient may use the musculoskeletal symptoms to explain why he or she just isn't getting along very well, thus using a mechanism of secondary gain like that of psychogenic rheumatism.

Again, the symptoms frequently don't come from specific body areas or follow usual nerve or muscle paths. The depression is general, so these syndromes will involve many parts of the body.

Similar symptoms occur with an inactive thyroid gland. Parkinson's disease is common in older people and can result in slowness and stiffness. Both thyroid disease and Parkinson's disease can be treated effectively, so it is important to recognize their presence.

PROGNOSIS

Because this is not an actual musculoskeletal condition, the prognosis is that of the depressive reaction. In a grief reaction, there is usually a return to normal after four to six months. With severe psychiatric depression, the period may be much longer.

TREATMENT

These syndromes are a signal to consider major lifestyle changes, even if the person's age is advanced. It is important to look forward to future events rather than only backward at what has gone before. New activities, new social groups, and new friends should be encouraged. It is a time for physical activity and for staying out of the house, even if such activities must be forced. Plant some young new trees and plan to attend the grandchildren's college graduations, even if they are only seven.

Medication may be required for treatment of the depression; such medication is often successful. On the other hand, the usual nonsteroidal musculoskeletal drugs should not be used. Drugs like Valium and codeine should be avoided. These drugs are themselves depressants, can aggravate symptoms, and may perpetuate the problem. Minor painkilling medications, such as acetaminophen (Tylenol) may be used but are unlikely to help a great deal. For further discussion, see Depression, **S5.**

If your problem is a general condition, proceed to Part II, page 103.

CHAPTER 11

The Connective-tissue Diseases
Not Quite Arthritis

Five diseases (systemic lupus erythematosus, rheumatoid arthritis, polymyositis, scleroderma, and polyarteritis) are frequently considered cousins and are grouped under the name *connective-tissue diseases.* These diseases are also sometimes called *autoimmune diseases* or *collagen-vascular diseases.* We have discussed three of these diseases (lupus, rheumatoid arthritis, and polymyositis) before. They can affect the joints or muscles, and the musculoskeletal part of the disease may be the major manifestation. But these conditions also affect other parts of the body. They involve several of the body organs. Arthritis is part of the picture, and a specialist in arthritis (rheumatologist) is often required for care or consultation.

Lupus (SLE): A Recap

Lupus is a disease of autoantibodies. The body's immune system seems to be producing too many antibodies, and some of these antibodies attack the tissues of the patient. The joints are one such tissue, but there are many others. Lupus is discussed beginning on page 26.

Rheumatoid Arthritis (RA): A Recap

Rheumatoid arthritis is listed here to indicate again that it is a systemic disease that affects many parts of the body. RA is discussed beginning on page 17.

Polymyositis (PM) and Dermatomyositis (DM): A Recap

These diseases of inflamed muscle can affect other parts of the body. They are discussed beginning on page 70.

Scleroderma

Scleroderma literally means "hard skin." The skin of a scleroderma patient, particularly over the fingers, arms, and sometimes face, can become stiff and bound down. The condition is due to a problem with the circulation through the small blood vessels, which eventually leads to scarring of the skin. If the skin becomes bound down and tight, the hands may become stiff. Because of the circulation problems, ulcers may develop in the fingertips.

Scleroderma, then, is not really arthritis. The problem is in the blood vessels and the skin and tissue around the joints, but it can lead to deformities not unlike those of arthritis. Actually, when you look at scleroderma joint tissues under the microscope, some signs of a true arthritis do appear.

The cause of scleroderma is not known. Current research suggests that problems in the smaller blood vessels result in damage to tissues. Earlier theories of too much scar tissue in the body are slowly being discarded, as are theories that antibodies, as in lupus, cause the disease.

FEATURES

Scleroderma patients usually have Raynaud's phenomenon, which can be the first sign of scleroderma. This phenomenon is a color change of the fingers, usually from pale to blue to red, after exposure to cold. Most people with Raynaud's phenomenon do not develop scleroderma, but a few do. *Acrosclerosis* is a medical term referring to hardening of the skin of the fingers and sometimes the toes. This occurs in most patients with scleroderma; sometimes there are calcium deposits beneath the skin as well. Hardening of the skin elsewhere is usually less impressive but may limit the ability to open the mouth or may cause some wrinkling around the eyes and mouth.

The scleroderma process can involve organs other than the skin. Most frequently the gastrointestinal tract is involved. The esophagus (gullet) can develop changes similar to those of the skin, and the swallowing wave can be interrupted. The stomach or small bowel may become dilated, and outpouchings of a special sort may develop in the colon. Scarring of the lower lungs may occur, and in a few patients the kidneys become abruptly involved, with high blood pressure and kidney failure.

Laboratory findings are not much help in diagnosis. X-rays may show calcium deposits in various places or may reveal the gastrointestinal tract problems noted above.

PROGNOSIS

The name does not help you much: *Progressive systemic sclerosis* (scleroderma) is often not progressive, not systemic, and not sclerosis. The name is misleading and unnecessarily ominous. Most patients do not have progressive courses. The disease will be active for a period of perhaps two years and then stabilize or even get better over the following years. It is not systemic in that only certain parts of the body are characteristically affected by scleroderma. Even these are not constant from patient to patient. Many patients have essentially just a mild skin condition. The condition is not truly sclerosis (which means "scarring") because scarring is only the accidental result of a problem of inadequate blood supply. The basic problem is inadequate flow through the small blood vessels.

The scleroderma patient frequently worries about the disease progressing to "mummylike" skin or, as it was once put, being "encased in a slowly shrinking, ever contracting, skin of steel." Fortunately, this doesn't happen. The skin involvement with scleroderma remains localized to the fingers, forearms, face, and neck in the overwhelming majority of patients, with perhaps some minor involvement of the toes and lower legs. With the exception of difficulty moving affected finger areas in advanced cases, scleroderma does not usually hamper a normal lifestyle.

Most people regard the appearance of calcium deposits as a bad sign. In fact, patients with calcinosis do better than other patients with scleroderma. In particular, patients with a syndrome of calcium deposits, Raynaud's phenomenon, esophageal swallowing problems, scleroderma involvement of the fingers, and little red spots called *telangiectasia* do particularly well. These patients are said to have the "CREST" syndrome, and they typically lead nearly normal lives. *CREST* stands for five disease manifestations: calcium deposits, Raynaud's color changes in the fingers with cold, esophageal problems (usually minor), scleroderma of the fingers, and telangiectatic red spots on the skin or lips.

Somewhere between 5% and 10% of patients with scleroderma develop a kidney problem. This is a serious medical complication and can lead to death in a short time. In recent years, life-saving medical treatment has been developed, and kidney dialysis and transplantation have been useful in patients who fail medical treatment. The sudden development of high blood pressure or of protein in the urine, a seizure, or decreased vision are worrisome signs in this disease, just as the presence of calcium beneath the skin is a good sign.

TREATMENT

The patient is the most important factor in successful adjustment to and recovery from this disease. For treatment of complications, however, the physician's role is crucial. It is essential that the patient's attitude toward life and the disease be positive. Good expectations work to increase blood flow through compromised blood vessels. The patient must actively exercise affected areas to stretch the skin and preserve full motion of the joints. Exercises such as placing the hand flat on a table and pressing until the fingers are straight, making a fist and then cocking the wrist to stretch the joint further, and so forth, should be repeated several times daily to improve circulation and maintain rotation.

Lifestyle should be as normal as possible. If symptoms of heartburn or stomach upset occur antacids are appropriate, and the doctor should be consulted about other treatment for *reflux esophagitis* (heartburn). Early treatment of heartburn can prevent some later difficulties with swallowing. Since the blood flow to the hands is less than perfect, good hand care is important. A cut on the fingers or fingertips may heal more slowly than in a person without the condition. Measures to keep the body warm to minimize Raynaud's phenomenon should include gloves as well as warmth for the trunk and neck areas that control the reflexes for blood flow to the fingers.

When complications occur, corticosteroid medications may be required for inflammation of the muscles. Medicines may be needed for high blood pressure and kidney disease. Antibiotics are successful for some of the gastrointestinal syndromes. Physician care and these powerful medicines can frequently help, but the day-to-day management of the uncomplicated disease depends on the patient.

If your problem is scleroderma, proceed to Part II, page 103.

Polyarteritis

"Inflammation of many arteries" is the problem with *polyarteritis* and actually represents the very meaning of the word. The arteries that supply blood to the body normally consist of an inner coat, a muscular middle layer, and an outer coat. Inflammation and destruction of all layers of these blood vessels occurs with polyarteritis. The organ for which the blood was sent does not receive the blood, and tissue damage occurs.

Several other diseases cause inflammation of the arteries, including polymyalgia rheumatica, described on page 68. The polyarteritis type of blood vessel inflammation, however, was the first discovered and is probably the most serious.

In recent years scientists have found the cause of some forms of polyarteritis. For example, the hepatitis virus can stimulate the body to form antibodies against the virus; the virus and the antibodies can then combine in the blood and lodge in the blood vessels. These *immune complexes* cause the inflammation that, in turn, causes damage to the vessel. In this case, polyarteritis is caused by a virus.

The key to understanding this complicated disease is its spotty involvement around the body. Various symptoms can be observed in various locations. But each problem has to result from inadequate blood supply caused by an attack on a particular blood vessel.

FEATURES

The lesions of polyarteritis are typically scattered but may come in "crops." In the skin they may consist of small spots with a central sore not much bigger than the head of a pin. The spot itself may be one-quarter to one-half inch (0.6 to 1.3 cm) in diameter. Each sore represents the interruption of blood flow through one small artery. In the lungs, X-rays can show pneumonias or even cavities within the lung that are the result of problems with the blood vessels. When the blood vessel that supplies a nerve is affected, the nerve ceases to work. There may be numbness or inability to use one particular muscle group. For example, there may be a "foot drop," in which the toes cannot be lifted upward and the foot slaps as the patient walks along. Involvement of the arteries can lead to kidney failure through inflammation of the blood vessels that supply blood to the kidney tissue.

In the laboratory there is little to assist in the diagnosis of polyarteritis. Often the fibrinogen level will be raised; this protein is part of the repair process for blood vessels. The platelet count may also be slightly raised and the sedimentation rate may be elevated.

Plain X-rays show little. In a difficult diagnostic case, an X-ray performed by injecting dye into the blood vessels of the abdomen may show little balloonlike aneurysms of the arteries.

A biopsy is the major technique for establishing a diagnosis of polyarteritis and is almost always required. A biopsy may be of the muscle, of the skin, the lung, or of other areas. The pathologist, looking at the biopsy under the microscope, can see the inflammation of the arteries and can establish the diagnosis.

PROGNOSIS

Until rather recently the prognosis for polyarteritis was not good. With current treatment, however, the prognosis is much better. Most patients return to a normal life after a sickness lasting some months, but many have to continue on medication with undesirable side effects for several years. Even now, despite excellent treatment, a few people die after only a few months of disease. Most of the time polyarteritis responds to treatment, but occasionally nothing seems to work.

TREATMENT

Prednisone (p. 137) is the major medication used and is given in high doses, with all of the resulting side effects. Immunosuppressive drugs (p. 149) are generally used along with the prednisone and have greatly decreased the rate of mortality from the disease. In both polyarteritis and another disease with inflammation in the arteries related to polyarteritis, *Wegener's granulomatosis,* treatment with both prednisone and an immunosuppressant agent is essential for a good result. Medications are tapered to lower doses over a period of several months to several years, and are eventually discontinued in many patients.

CHAPTER 12

Osteoporosis

Brittle Bones

Osteoporosis is a bone disease in which the bones lose calcium, become more brittle, and break more easily. While anyone can have osteoporosis, it is most common in elderly people, particularly women. Because of osteoporosis, one in five women breaks a hip before the age of 75. Fractures of the spine, resulting in pain, decrease in height, and a forward deformity of the spine (dowager's hump) are even more common. Inactivity makes osteoporosis worse.

Although the best protection from osteoporosis is prevention, we now have some effective treatments. As with all kinds of arthritis and rheumatism, consistent good health practices are crucial. This starts with a lifestyle that excludes smoking and drinking too much alcohol. The following pages outline the healthy habits that are useful in preventing and dealing with osteoporosis.

Dietary Calcium

Our bones cannot maintain their strength unless our bodies regularly receive an adequate supply of calcium. Recently the National Institutes of Health (NIH) Consensus Development Conference on optimal calcium intake concluded that millions of Americans are not getting nearly enough calcium in their diets and that the official recommended daily allowance (RDA) for calcium may not be adequate for some age groups. Table 12.1 shows the recommended amounts for different ages.

To bring your calcium intake up to 800 or 1,000 mg, eat two or three servings of milk products a day (nonfat milk is best) and regularly include other calcium-rich foods in your meals (see Table 12.2). Also try to moderate the amount of salt and meat you eat; excessive amounts of sodium

TABLE 12.1 *Recommended Calcium Intake*

Age Group	*Optimal Daily Intake (in milligrams)*	*Recommended Daily Allowance (in milligrams)*
Infants birth to 6 months	400 (250 if nursing)	400
Infants 6 months to 1 year	600	600
Children 1 to 10 years old	800	800
Teenagers	1,200 to 1,500	1,200
Men		
20 to 50	800	800
51 to 65	1,000	800
Over 65	1,500	800
Women		
20 to 50	1,000	800
Over 50	1,500 (1,000 if taking estrogen)	800
Pregnant and nursing	Additional 400	1,200

or meat can increase your need for calcium. If you don't tolerate milk products well, you probably need the calcium supplements described below.

Table 12.2 gives you a good idea of the types of food that are relatively rich in calcium. Notice that you can get significant quantities of calcium without drinking milk. Yogurts, cheeses, and hot cereals made with milk all supply calcium. Canned salmon, mackerel, and sardines are excellent sources of calcium *if* you eat the soft bones.

SUPPLEMENTAL CALCIUM

It is better to get calcium from your foods than to rely on calcium supplements. But if you cannot eat two or more servings of dairy products every day, or if you want to take in more than 1,000 mg of calcium, supplements can provide practical help.

In general, choose a supplement that contains between 500 and 1,000 mg (50 to 100% of the RDA) of elemental calcium. *Elemental calcium* means the actual amount of calcium in the pill. Take one or two full doses a day, depending on your needs—not more.

As Table 12.3 illustrates, the elemental calcium in a supplement can come from any of several different calcium compounds. Less expensive store-brand supplements are usually fine; use the product that suits you

TABLE 12.2 *Food Sources of Calcium*

Food	*Amount*	*Calcium (approximate)*
Low-fat and nonfat milk products		
Nonfat milk	1 cup (235 ml)	300 mg
Low-fat milk (1% fat)	1 cup (235 ml)	300 mg
Low-fat milk (2% fat)	1 cup (235 ml)	295 mg
Nonfat dry milk powder	3 tbsp (45 ml)	280 mg
Nonfat yogurt (plain)	1 cup (235 ml)	450 mg
Low-fat yogurt (plain)	1 cup (235 ml)	415 mg
Low-fat cottage cheese (2% fat)	1 cup (235 ml)	155 mg
Part-skim ricotta cheese	1/2 cup (120 ml)	335 mg
Part-skim mozzarella	2 oz (56 g)	365 mg
Whole milk products		
Whole milk (3.5% fat)	1 cup (235 ml)	290 mg
Whole-milk yogurt (plain)	1 cup (235 ml)	275 mg
Swiss cheese	1 oz (28 g)	270 mg
Processed Swiss cheese	1 oz (28 g)	220 mg
Cheddar cheese	1 oz (28 g)	205 mg
Processed American cheese	1 oz (28 g)	125 mg
Ice milk (hard, not soft-serve)	1 cup (235 ml)	175 mg
Ice cream (regular, 10% fat)	1 cup (235 ml)	175 mg
Ice cream (rich, 16% fat)	1 cup (235 ml)	150 mg
Other calcium-rich foods		
Almonds	1 oz (28 g)	75 mg
Broccoli (boiled)	1 cup (235 ml)	180 mg
Corn tortilla	1	40 mg
Great northern beans (boiled)	1 cup (235 ml)	120 mg
Kale (boiled)	1 cup (235 ml)	95 mg
Navy beans (boiled)	1 cup (235 ml)	130 mg
Pinto beans (boiled)	1 cup (235 ml)	80 mg
Tofu (soybean curd)	1/2 cup (120 ml)	130 mg
Canned jack mackerel (including bones)	1/2 cup (120 ml)	230 mg
Canned salmon (including bones)	3 oz (84 g)	190 mg
Canned sardines (including bones)	1 oz (28 g)	85 mg

For most people, low-fat and nonfat dairy products are better choices than full-fat products.

TABLE 12.3 *Supplemental Calcium*

Sources of Supplemental Calcium	*Elemental Calcium Content*
Calcium carbonate (in oyster-shell calcium, BioCal, Caltrate 600, OsCal, Tums)	40%
Calcium citrate (in CitraCal)	21%
Calcium lactate (available in store-brand products)	13%

best. Sometimes inexpensive calcium tablets won't dissolve in your stomach, however, so try this test. Put a tablet in half a glass of water for 30 minutes. It should become shaggy and partly dissolve. If not, fill the glass the rest of the way with vinegar, stir gently, and wait another half hour. If the tablet is still not dissolved, it is not a good product for you.

MYTHS ABOUT CALCIUM

- **Calcium causes bone spurs.** Maintaining a calcium intake of 800 to 1,500 mg a day (or even much higher) will not cause bone spurs.
- **Calcium causes kidney stones.** While it is prudent to avoid calcium intakes that exceed 2,000 mg a day, consuming a total of 800 to 1,500 mg a day is unlikely to lead to kidney stones. If you have had kidney stones in the past, you should check with your doctor before starting a calcium supplement. Otherwise, just be sure to drink plenty of fluids whenever you take a calcium tablet.
- **Calcium causes constipation.** Large doses of calcium can cause constipation in some people. But the problem generally can be avoided by drinking plenty of fluids and eating foods high in fiber.

Hormones

Calcium by itself will not stop bone loss. The body needs a stimulus to absorb the calcium and to get it into the bone. The best stimuli are estrogen therapy for postmenopausal women and adequate weight-bearing exercise for everybody. The use of hormones such as estrogen after menopause has long been a topic of controversy. This is a subject every woman should discuss with her physician. The following discussion is to help you understand some of the issues.

ESTROGEN

There are two female hormones, estrogen and progestin. These hormones are normally secreted during the menstrual cycle. After menopause their levels fall greatly. Taking supplemental estrogen after menopause protects against osteoporosis. However, it is believed by some to increase the likelihood of endometrial cancer (cancer of the lining of the uterus) or even breast cancer. When progesterone is taken with the estrogen, this risk is greatly reduced and there is generally no problem with menstrual spotting as may occur with estrogen alone. The greatest health benefit from estrogen or estrogen/progestin is a nearly 50% reduction in the risk of heart disease, which far outweighs any risks. These hormones also help prevent hot flashes, vaginal dryness, dementia, and skin wrinkling. The decision to take no hormone, one hormone (either estrogen or progestin), or a combination of the two is a personal one and should be discussed with a physician. Most physicians now recommend estrogens for postmenopausal women.

OTHER TREATMENTS

Calcitonin

An approved alternative to estrogen-replacement therapy for treatment of osteoporosis is salmon calcitonin. Calcitonin can actually help build back strong bones, not just slow down the process of bone loss. The major drawback to the treatment has been its expense and the necessity for patients to learn how to self-administer injections. The medication may cause transient flushing and nausea in about 20% of patients. Calcitonin administration by nasal spray is now possible and is considerably easier.

Biphosphonates

Etidronate (Didronel) was the first of a class of drugs called biphosphonates, followed by Clodronate. These "first-generation" biphosphonates are usually given for a two-week period every three months (cyclic therapy) since they don't work if given continuously. These drugs have been shown to produce a small increase in bone density and to decrease the frequency of spine fractures. Because biphosphonates are poorly absorbed, they must be taken on an empty stomach and only with water. Long-term efficacy is still under investigation.

Second- and third-generation biphosphonates are now available, led by alendronate (Fosamax) and including pamidronate, tiludronate, and ibandronate (all second-generation), and residronate (third-generation). These can be taken continuously and decrease the risk of spinal fractures by 50 to 90%, even in persons who have already had a fracture. These drugs can irritate the stomach so they are best taken in the morning with a glass of warm water. The third-generation residronate causes less stomach irritation.

Vitamin D

Vitamin D comes with sunlight and diet. If you are usually indoors and malnourished, supplementation (as with a multivitamin) may be a good idea.

Fluoride

Low-dose fluoride (2–5 mg per day) is felt to be helpful by some physicians; high doses can actually cause brittle bones. Slow-release fluoride (25 mg twice a day for 12 months followed by 2 months off) has been shown to increase bone mass and decrease vertebral fractures but is not yet available in the United States.

Experimental Treatments

Parathyroid fragments and growth factors are under study and appear promising.

Exercise

Weight-bearing exercise is very, very important in maintaining strong bones. The body reacts to such exercise by increasing the calcium content and, thus, the strength of the bones. Walking is the best such exercise. If at all possible, walk half a mile to a mile (1 to 1.6 km) a day. If this is unrealistic for you, remember that even a little weight-bearing exercise is important. Do as much as you can. Recent research has shown that women need to walk four miles (6 km) a week to get maximal exercise benefit for osteoporosis prevention. This includes all the walking we do in our daily lives. (Note: Swimming is *not* a weight-bearing exercise.)

Preventing Falls

Unfortunately it is not always possible to prevent osteoporosis or undo damage already done. Remember, osteoporosis by itself does not cause pain. The pain comes from fractures in the spine or other bones. Thus, avoiding falls is very important to prevent broken bones. Following are a few hints:

- Avoid area rugs—they are slippery and have a bad habit of tripping the unwary.
- Be sure that all stairs have a secure railing that is easy to grasp.

- If advised to do so by a health professional, use a cane, stick, or walker. These can be real bone savers.
- Even if you don't usually use a cane, consider using one for getting up at night. This is a time when most of us may easily lose our balance, and a cane can help prevent bad spills.
- Watch for uneven walks, curbs, floors, and so on.
- Move the phone to a convenient place so you won't trip over the cord.
- Wear shoes that give good support.
- Use step stools that are stable and in good repair.
- Use nonskid mats in the bathtub and shower, and on the bathroom floor. Install permanent grab bars on the wall or edge of the tub.
- If you are unsteady on your feet, sit on a stool with nonskid feet when showering or bathing.
- Have light switches at the top and bottom of all stairs.
- Be careful not to hold your breath when you are on the toilet. This can cause you to pass out and fall.

Summary: Preventing and Treating Osteoporosis

There are five things you can do to help prevent and treat osteoporosis:

1. Make positive lifestyle changes: stop smoking, reduce alcohol consumption.
2. Do some weight-bearing exercise every day.
3. Using diet or a combination of diet and supplements, take adequate calcium.
4. If advised by your physician, take estrogen, progestin, a combination of these hormones, biphosphonates, vitamin D, or sodium fluoride.
5. Make your home and other surroundings fall-safe.

For more information on osteoporosis there is an excellent new book by Dr. Nancy Lane, *The Osteoporosis Book: A Guide for Patients and Their Families* (New York: Oxford University Press, 1999).

PART II

Managing Your Arthritis

CHAPTER 13

Treatment Begins at Home

Self-management of arthritis should be guided by common sense. Self-management is as important as medical management, and you need to understand the effects of your lifestyle on your disease. There are three major factors that you may be neglecting. Let's consider these first, and then proceed to some general conclusions.

The Major Lifestyle Factors

YOUR BODY'S DEFENSES

First, revere the defense mechanisms of the body; they are many and wonderful. The body reacts to anything that disturbs its health by means of these mechanisms. In our society many people have forgotten just how useful they are. The cough that clears foreign material or bacteria from our lungs, the diarrhea that helps carry the food toxin outside of our body, the runny nose that takes the virus outside where it can do no harm—all are essential to the maintenance of good health. Yet, curiously, we often consider defense mechanisms to be diseases.

An important defense mechanism is *pain.* Pain can tell you that you are overusing an injured joint or are interfering with the natural healing of a sprained ligament. Animals do very well with arthritis and muscle problems because they let the internal doctor, pain, guide their activities.

If your pain improves with exercise, then gently increasing an exercise program makes sense. If pain gets worse or occurs after exercise, that's a signal for backing off from that particular activity. Pain isn't pleasant. You don't need to like it. But it can help you. Don't blunt the pain sensation with pain medications if you can get by without the medications. You need the advice given by this unpleasant sensation.

Fatigue is another defense mechanism. Fatigue is the body's way of telling you that it needs rest, and you ought to listen to this "doctor" as well. Pain and fatigue provide you with a constant stream of advice about what you should be doing.

EXERCISE

Second, remember that exercise has far more benefits than drawbacks for the person with arthritis. The bones react to exercise and to bearing weight by growing stronger. The body absorbs more calcium, deposits it in the bones, and creates thicker and sturdier support structures. Exercise builds the muscles and increases muscle tone. This creates support across the joints and helps to stabilize joints. The tendons, as well as the ligaments, gain strength when they are used. Each of these tissues gets weaker when it is not used.

The cartilage of the joint is a most interesting tissue. This gristle does not have a blood supply. It gets oxygen and nourishment and gets rid of waste products by compression—fluid is squeezed into the joint space, then is removed and replenished. The health of the cartilage depends on motion, because without motion there is no nourishment of the cartilage. Even a few weeks in a plaster cast may result in cartilage degeneration. In contrast, marathon runners and others who subject their cartilage to great stress throughout life tend not to have excessive degeneration of the cartilage.

Exercise also gives major psychological benefits. It is an excellent way to fight anxiety and depression. The physical tiredness induced by exercise increases the depth of the sleep period, which in turn improves energy and vigor the following day. Further, the social interactions encouraged by exercise are themselves very healthy.

There is one drawback to exercising with arthritis. If the arthritis is an inflammatory synovitis (such as rheumatoid arthritis), exercise of the inflamed part may make the inflammation temporarily worse. For this reason there is some controversy among doctors about the proper role of rest and exercise. The consensus is that exercise is necessary for all patients with all forms of arthritis. With active synovitis, exercise should be limited (while the active inflammation persists) to levels that do not greatly increase the pain and inflammation. There are always techniques, such as isometrics, which allow exercise without increasing inflammation.

Rest does just the opposite of exercise. It does reduce inflammation when inflammation is present, but it increases calcium loss from bone, allows the muscles and tendons to weaken, and fails to nourish the cartilage. It has the psychological disadvantage of encouraging dependency.

YOUR GOALS FOR LIFE

Third, decide what you want to accomplish. Lifestyle is your own choice. But the clock is ticking. You would like to increase the days of full functioning in your life. If you put off the challenge posed by your arthritis to "when you feel better," you may never get around to it. Or when you finally do decide to start a program of active living, your muscles, bones, tendons, and habits may be so out of shape that getting back into condition for normal activity will be a long-term process. When you consider what you want to accomplish, you may find that some adjustments are necessary. For the most part, however, you can do whatever you set out to do.

Now, a caution about doctors. We can't always tell how much you hurt. We have trouble telling exactly how tired and fatigued you are. We tend to give you arbitrary rules, good for most people but perhaps not quite right for you. Studies show that you don't take our advice about activity and lifestyle very seriously anyhow, so these decisions are largely up to you and your common sense. Let's test the principles above on some of the questions most commonly asked.

Should I Work?

Sure, if you can. Some physical occupations may require that you make adjustments because they put too much stress across joints and increase pain and discomfort. Or if your arthritis is severe, you may be incapable of doing them. But there is usually an alternative job or better job that you can do very well. If you work, you may have less energy left for your home life, and you may have to simplify your home life in one way or another—a smaller house, domestic help, or the like. But this can also be true for people without arthritis. The payoffs for working are satisfaction, productivity, pride, and money. And if you don't blunt your pain response with too much pain medication, it's difficult to hurt yourself or injure your joints, because the arthritis process itself will prevent that.

How Much Exercise?

Work up to it. Listen for the pain message. Go slow. The principles of conditioning are well understood by coaches and by good athletes. They consist of regular exercise, slowly increased to the desired level. Some setbacks are to be expected during an exercise program. Don't let them scare you off. They are not permanent. Keep at it.

What Kind of Exercise?

There are many different kinds of exercise and, depending on your problems, you will want to mix them in differing degrees; more specific discussions appear in Part III. Exercise as a regular part of your daily activities, gently graded, builds muscle and heart tone, strengthens ligaments, decreases anxiety, and does a lot of other good things. Therapeutic exercises directed at problems with specific areas of the body can increase the motion at joints or strengthen specific regions, such as the upper leg muscles.

Here are three "dos" and a "don't":

- *Do* be regular and slowly progressive with your exercise program.
- *Do* stretching and range-of-motion exercises on a regular basis. Affected joints should be stretched to the limits of discomfort several times daily in order to prevent permanent stiffness at the joints.
- *Do* smooth regular exercises with many repetitions. Examples of such exercises are swimming, bicycling, and walking. No tremendously strenuous actions are required by these exercises. They can be gradually increased, and you can stop them at any time you feel tired or hurt too much.
- *Don't* do high-tension exercises requiring forces across the joints. Weight lifting, ball squeezing, and so forth place more stress across the injured joint than the joint needs. Intermediate-tension exercises include tennis, bowling, and golf, which require strength and jerky movements to varying degrees. Bicycling puts stress across the knee and should be done with care if the knees are sore or swollen. If you ride a bicycle or a stationary bicycle, make sure the seat is high enough so that the knees do not have to bend to more than a right angle.

The Arthritis Helpbook provides an assortment of flexibility and strengthening exercises, plus advice on finding the right exercise program for you.

When Should I Rest?

When you are tired. The dilemma of rest versus overexercise causes misunderstanding. Doctors usually recommend both rest and exercise, and patients perceive this as a contradiction. Actually the two modes should alternate. When you are tired, listen to the fatigue message coming from your body. Don't be afraid to get a little bit tired, but if you require a nap midday or a nap after work, then take it. Try to keep the rest periods relatively short. Naps during the day may take away from your night sleep. By doing too much napping during the day you can get into a vicious cycle that has you feeling tired all the time. Between rests, be active.

What About Diet?

Diet and arthritis. This curious theme repeats itself in dozens of quack remedies. Every patient with arthritis at some point wonders if the disease is the result of some improper eating habit or if the disease would disappear if correct foods were eaten. The central question, "Why did I get arthritis?", seldom has a good answer, so we tend to accept any answer at all.

Quacks have suggested that cod-liver oil, vitamins, mineral supplements, vegetarian diets, honey and vinegar, fresh fruits and laxatives, low fat, high fat, low protein, high protein, and every other imaginable combination of foods will cure arthritis. Each diet contradicts the others.

There is no special diet for arthritis. The best-known relationship between food and arthritis is with gout, where a diet heavy in purines will increase the chances of an attack. Patients with gout should avoid sweetbreads, liver, kidney, and brain, since these foods are very rich in purines. Fish oil capsules have been found to decrease inflammation slightly in rheumatoid arthritis, but this treatment has not become very popular.

If you think about it, you know that diet is not the answer. You didn't eat differently from anyone else before you had your arthritis. You also know that there are many kinds of arthritis and that there cannot be a single cause or cure for all kinds. It is tempting to accept a simple answer to a complicated problem, but it just isn't that easy. Keep your common sense active.

Weight control is important for the prevention and the treatment of many kinds of arthritis, and in this sense diet is very important. This subject is discussed in Overweight (Obesity), **S6.**

A balanced, moderate diet is part of the good health habits you want to develop. The body needs raw materials of various sorts for daily work and for repair. Foods from each of the major groups, together with vitamins, minerals, and fluid, are all required, but not in excess. The diet good for your general health is good for your arthritis. We recommend diets low in total calories, low in saturated fats, low in salt, and high in unrefined carbohydrates (that is, the natural kind found in whole grains, beans, fruits, and vegetables). In *Take Care of Yourself* we discuss your diet for health in more detail, and in *The Arthritis Helpbook* we discuss the special needs of people with arthritis.

What About Climate?

Some people with arthritis can forecast the weather. An approaching low-pressure system, with a falling barometer, causes an increase in pain and stiffness in such patients. Scientists have tested this phenomenon in pressure chambers, and it is indeed true.

So should you move to Arizona? The warmth of the desert sun might bake out some of those aches, and the high-pressure weather systems over the desert will minimize the pains caused by changing barometric pressure.

Sometimes. The course of arthritis is not really changed by living in desert areas. Comfort is improved for some patients but not for others. Is slight improvement in comfort worth the disruption entailed by a move to a new place? Often it is not. If you are thinking seriously about such a move, take an extended vacation in the new place first. If you are going to feel better on the desert, improvement will be evident within a few weeks. If the combination of vacation and sun doesn't help very much, a permanent move is not a good idea.

Expectations

Your expectations are the key to how well you will do with your arthritis. Franklin Roosevelt declared during the Depression that "the only thing we have to fear is fear itself." Although this phrase has become trite from overuse, for the patient with arthritis, nothing is truer.

Expectations for individual patients vary. Realistic expectations, however, are almost always good. The patient who assumes the worst is in big trouble. Such patients often get into a cycle much like the following: The patient gives up a job because of anticipated future disability; he or she takes a dependent role at home; self-image is decreased and personal pride diminished; the patient uses the disease to manipulate others and loses friends; the patient never leaves home so no new friends are made; and a downward spiral into passive isolation and unhappiness continues.

A handicap, if you have one from arthritis, is just that. Eyeglasses, a hearing aid, a wooden leg, a crutch. Arthritis, heart disease, cancer, stroke. There are two kinds of people: those who have a handicap now, and those who are going to have one.

Illness is a human experience. Many patients become finer persons because of the insights, the sensitivity, and the empathy induced by living with a chronic illness. The ability to understand the problems of others, to offer hope and help, and to serve as a model for those around you may be enhanced by the presence of arthritis.

It is not easy to see any positive side to a disability and to escape depression and anger. In the first months of a long disease it may be impossible. If your arthritis is serious, it may represent the greatest challenge of your life. Meeting the challenge can be your greatest satisfaction. Christiaan Barnard performed the first heart transplant operation and innumerable cardiac surgical procedures *with* rheumatoid arthritis. Rosalind Russell maintained a vigorous public life of tremendous public service while battling severe rheumatoid arthritis. Jerry Walsh retired from professional baseball because of rheumatoid arthritis and spent an energetic life crusading against quack treatments and for sound management of arthritis. Byron Janis maintained a brilliant career as a concert pianist despite psoriatic arthritis involving the hands. The list goes on.

Think forward. Make plans. Set goals. Carry them out. You need a bit more will and determination and self-discipline than others. But the future still can be yours.

CHAPTER 14

The Drug Scene
Medicines to Reduce Pain and Inflammation

Recently there has been an unprecedented explosion of new and different treatments for arthritis. Some are safer than previously available alternatives, some use entirely new approaches to arthritis relief, and some give better results for some—but not all—patients. The period beginning in 1998 has brought the most exciting wave of new arthritis treatments ever seen. This is good news for patients, but both doctors and patients need to learn about the new drugs and how to use them wisely.

Knowing all about your drugs is important, but it is not easy. Drugs have complex effects on your body, some good and some bad, and a full explanation from your doctor always takes lots of time. Unfortunately that time is not always available in the modern doctor visit, which is all too brief. The interview with your doctor is an intensive experience, and detailed discussion of prescribed treatment is often neglected. Little time is spent on the important subject of how to use your medications correctly. In chapters 14, 15, and 16, the discussions you've been having with your physician are repeated. Read the ones you need. Reread those you've forgotten.

There are four major types of arthritis medications. First, there are drugs that both moderate inflammation and reduce pain (NSAIDs). Second, there are corticosteroid hormone anti-inflammatory medications. Third, there are strongly anti-inflammatory disease modifying drugs (DMARDs), which improve the overall course of an inflammatory arthritis such as rheumatoid arthritis. And fourth, there are drugs that are analgesic only, directed at relieving pain. We discuss the first two types in this chapter, and the third and fourth in Chapter 15 and Chapter 16, respectively.

Anti-inflammatory Medications

INFLAMMATION

The pain, swelling, and joint destruction caused by many kinds of arthritis are a result of inflammation around the joint. Many important arthritis medicines are intended to reduce inflammation. Yet inflammation also is part of the body's normal healing process. When injured, the body increases blood flow to the injured area and sends inflammatory cells to repair the wounded tissue and to kill bacterial invaders. The inflammation causes the area to be warm, red, tender, and often swollen. To understand the potential problems of drugs that reduce inflammation, it is important to recognize first that inflammation is a normal process and often can be helpful rather than harmful.

In osteoarthritis there is little inflammation, or the inflammation may be necessary for the healing process. But in rheumatoid arthritis, psoriatic arthritis, ankylosing spondylitis, and other inflammatory forms of arthritis, the inflammation itself causes damage; thus, suppression of the inflammation can be helpful in treatment. You don't always want anti-inflammatory drugs just because you have arthritis: in osteoarthritis, often no; in rheumatoid arthritis, you want strong ones, usually DMARDs.

NONSTEROIDAL ANTI-INFLAMMATORY DRUGS (NSAIDs) AND ASPIRIN

The first NSAID was aspirin, introduced in 1898. Chewing of willow bark, which contains salicylate, to relieve pain had been practiced for several hundred years before that. The newer NSAIDs began to arrive in the mid-1960s when Indocin, Motrin, Naprosyn, Tolectin, and Nalfon became available. Many, many NSAIDs have been introduced since. Some work better than others for particular patients. Some have more side effects than others. In low doses these drugs are analgesic; that is, they relieve pain. In higher doses they also reduce inflammation.

These drugs have important roles beyond the treatment of arthritis. Low-dose aspirin is effective in preventing heart attacks. It appears that some NSAIDs are useful in preventing colon cancer, and some may even slow the development of Alzheimer's disease.

NSAIDs work by blocking the enzyme cyclo-oxygenase (COX), which stimulates inflammation. The major side effects of these drugs come from the same blocking of the COX enzyme. The drugs deplete a protective chemical, prostaglandin, in the wall of the stomach and other parts of the gastrointestinal (GI) tract. As a result, ulcers can form, and these can cause serious bleeding from the stomach as well as other complications. Because NSAIDs are so widely used, over 100,000 hospitalizations in the United States and over 10,000 deaths each year are caused by the gastrointestinal side effects of these drugs. The people most likely to get these side effects are older; more disabled; taking higher doses of the drugs; taking the drugs for longer periods; and taking prednisone at the same time. They also have had previous side effects with drugs of this class.

Since recognition of the problem of "NSAID gastropathy" some ten years ago, largely as a result of research by our group, there has been a search for less toxic NSAIDs and for treatments that can block side effects. This search has been largely successful. First, misoprostil (Cytotec) was introduced. Misoprostil itself is a prostaglandin and replaces the lost prostaglandin in the stomach wall, preventing many problems. Unfortunately, it often causes diarrhea. After misoprostil, less toxic NSAIDs were discovered. These were less acidic or were somewhat safer for other reasons. Rheumatologists now often use lower NSAID doses or use Tylenol instead.

The most recent and most important approach toward safer NSAIDs has come from a new scientific discovery. The enzyme COX has been found to be two enzymes, now called COX-1 and COX-2. The side effects come almost entirely from blockage of the COX-1 enzyme, and the desired anti-inflammatory effects from blockage of COX-2. New drugs, called selective COX-2 inhibitors, preserve most of the desired effects while eliminating most of the undesired ones. Actually the new drugs would be better termed "COX-1 sparing" drugs, since these drugs are *not* more powerful anti-inflammatory agents than older drugs. Their effectiveness is about the same. The advantage of the newer drugs is greater safety.

NSAIDs AND SIDE EFFECTS

It used to be thought that all NSAIDs had about the same toxicity. Then research, first by our research group and later by others, proved that there were big differences in the frequency of side effects with different NSAIDs. Table 14.1 lists NSAIDs, grouped by the frequency of serious gastrointestinal (GI) side effects. The individual drugs are discussed in more detail later in this chapter. Misoprostil, which can be combined with any of the NSAIDs to improve safety, is discussed under Arthrotec. The groupings of Table 14.1 are consistent with recent research but still are not completely proven. On average, the most toxic NSAIDs will be three or more times as toxic as the least toxic. Costs are estimated from our data, from the manufacturer's data in some cases, and from the formulary listings of a major national health plan. Within groupings, the drugs are listed in alphabetical order.

If you are taking one of the more toxic NSAIDs, or even one of the moderately toxic ones, you might want to discuss with your doctor whether a less toxic NSAID might work just as well. Remember, all drugs can cause side effects, and the safety of any drug is only relative compared with others. Different people respond better or worse to different drugs.

TABLE 14.1 *NSAID Toxicity for Serious Gastrointestinal (GI) Problems*

Nonsteroidal Anti-inflammatory Drug (NSAID)	*Estimated Cost (branded/generic)*
Least Toxic NSAIDs	
Arthrotec (diclofenac and misoprostil)	$$$/–
ASA (aspirin) less than 2600 mg/day*	$/$
Celebrex (celecoxib)	$$$/–
Lodine (etodolac)	$$/–
Mobic (meloxicam)	$$/–
Motrin (ibuprofen)*	$$/$
Relafen (nabumetone)	$$/–
Salsalate (salicylate)*	$$/$$
Trilisate (trisalicylate)*	$$/$$
Vioxx (rofecoxib)	$$$/–
Moderately Toxic NSAIDs	
Clinoril (sulindac)	$$/$$
Daypro (oxaprozin)	$$/–
Dolobid (diflunisal)	$$/$
Naprosyn (naproxen)*	$$/$
Orudis (ketoprofen)*	$$/$
Voltaren (diclofenac)	$$$/$$
Most Toxic NSAIDs	
Ansaid (flurbiprofen)	$$/–
Feldene (piroxicam)	$$/$
Indocin (indomethacin)	$/$
Meclomen (meclofenamate)	$$/$$
Nalfon (fenoprofen)	$$/$
Tolectin (tolmetin)	$$/$$

$$$ most expensive
$$ moderately expensive
$ least expensive

* available over-the-counter
– not available in generic product

NOTE: Tylenol (acetaminophen), which is analgesic only, would be among the least toxic and least expensive medications.

Here are some hints about NSAID side effects. Lower doses of these drugs are always less toxic than higher doses. If you have a serious medical problem such as heart failure, liver disease, or kidney disease, the drugs are likely to be more toxic, and even lower doses may be needed. Generic forms of these drugs are similar in both effectiveness and toxicity to brand-name drugs; they are much less expensive, as can be seen in the table. The more recently introduced drugs are more expensive than the earlier ones, and generic drugs usually are the least expensive. The claim "as safe as aspirin" is misleading; all of these drugs—including aspirin—need to be used carefully and with respect. When two or more drugs are taken, there can be drug interactions that cause other side effects, as with additional toxicity when prednisone is taken at the same time as and interferes with blood-thinning medicines such as Coumadin. If you are taking other medicines, you should ask your doctor if any drug interactions with NSAIDs are likely.

What follows in the remainder of this chapter are general recommendations. If your doctor's advice differs, then listen to your doctor. He or she is most familiar with your specific needs. The cautions listed are those known at the time of this writing and are subject to changes that your doctor may know about. But if you receive advice that doesn't make sense according to the principles outlined in this section, don't hesitate to ask questions or get another opinion.

Aspirin and Other Salicylates

ACETYLSALICYLIC ACID (aspirin)

PURPOSE

To relieve pain; to reduce inflammation.

INDICATIONS

Pain relief for osteoarthritis, rheumatoid arthritis, and local conditions such as bursitis. Anti-inflammatory agent for rheumatoid arthritis if taken in high doses.

DOSAGE

For pain, two 5-grain tablets (5 grains equals 325 mg) every four hours as needed. For anti-inflammatory action, three to four tablets, four to six times daily (with medical supervision if these doses are continued for longer than one week). The time to maximum effect is thirty minutes to one hour for pain and one to three weeks for the anti-inflammatory action.

SIDE EFFECTS

Common effects include nausea, vomiting, ringing in the ears, and decreased hearing. Each of these is reversible within a few hours if the drug dosage is decreased. Allergic reactions are rare but include development of nasal polyps and wheezing. With an overdose of aspirin there is very rapid and heavy breathing, and there can even be unconsciousness and coma. Be sure to keep aspirin (and all medications) out of the reach of children.

Aspirin has some predictable effects that occur in just about everyone. Blood loss through the bowel occurs in almost all persons who take aspirin, because the blood clotting function is decreased, the stomach is irritated, and aspirin acts as a minor blood-thinning agent. Up to 10% of those taking very high doses of aspirin will have some abnormalities in the function of the liver; although these are seldom noticed by the person taking aspirin they can be identified by blood tests. Since serious liver damage does not occur, routine blood tests to check for this complication usually are not required. Hospitalization for gastrointestinal hemorrhage occurs in about 1% of people taking full doses for one year.

Aspirin is not recommended for children with influenza, chicken pox, or high fevers because of the possibility of a rare liver and brain complication called Reye syndrome.

SPECIAL HINTS

Aspirin remains an important drug for treatment of arthritis. If you note ringing in the ears or a decrease in your hearing, then decrease the dose of aspirin. Your dose is just a little bit too high for the best result. Some people develop nasal polyps or wheezing with salicylates; if you are one of those people, these drugs are not for you.

If you notice nausea, an upset stomach, or vomiting, there are a variety of things you can do. First, try spreading out the dose with more frequent use of smaller numbers of pills. Perhaps instead of taking four tablets four times a day, you might take three tablets five or six times a day. Second, try taking the aspirin after meals or after an antacid, which will coat the stomach and provide some protection. Third, you can change brands and see if the nausea is related to the particular brand of aspirin you are using. Fourth, you can try coated aspirin (Ecotrin). These tablets are not always absorbed well but are often effective in protecting the stomach and decreasing nausea. Although it is a nuisance, you often can get good relief from the nausea by taking a suspension of aspirin rather than the tablet. Put the aspirin in a half glass of water and swirl it until the aspirin particles are suspended in the water. Fill another glass half full of water, drink the suspended aspirin, and wash it down with the other glass of water. This is an effective and inexpensive way to avoid nausea once you get used to the taste. You can also mix the aspirin with juice or milk.

Keep track of your aspirin intake and always tell your doctor exactly how much you are taking. Aspirin is so familiar that sometimes we forget we are taking a drug. Be as careful with aspirin as you would be with any other drug. In particular you may want to ask your doctor about interactions with the newer anti-inflammatory agents, with probenecid, or with blood-thinning drugs. Pay special attention to your stomach. So many drugs cause irritation to the stomach lining that you run the risk of adding insult to injury. Two drugs that irritate the stomach lining may be more than twice as dangerous as one. Again, the fewer medications taken at one time the better. Every time you talk to a doctor, be sure to describe all the drugs you are taking, not just your arthritis drugs. It is wise to keep a list of all the drugs you take and have it ready to show any doctor you visit, including your dentist.

DISALCID (salsalate)

500 mg round, aqua, scored, film-coated tablet
500 mg aqua and white capsule
750 mg capsule-shaped, aqua, scored, film-coated tablet

PURPOSE

To relieve pain; to reduce inflammation.

INDICATIONS

For mild pain relief of osteoarthritis and in local conditions. As an anti-inflammatory agent for synovitis or attachment arthritis, as in rheumatoid arthritis and ankylosing spondylitis.

DOSAGE

For pain, one or two 750 mg tablets every 12 hours. Each 750 mg Disalcid tablet is equivalent in salicylate content to about two and a half normal-sized (325 mg) aspirin tablets. Occasionally higher doses may be needed. For pain, the maximum effect is reached in two hours; one to three weeks are required for anti-inflammatory action to take full effect.

SIDE EFFECTS

Side effects include nausea, vomiting, ringing in the ears, and decreased hearing, but are not common. Each of these is reversible within a few hours if the drug dosage is decreased. Allergic reactions are rare but may include development of nasal polyps and wheezing. With an overdose of any salicylate there can be very heavy and rapid breathing, which can lead to unconsciousness and coma.

Disalcid is being used more frequently in arthritis because it appears to be less toxic to the stomach than most other NSAIDs, although definitive data are not available. Additionally, Disalcid has less effect on the platelets, so there is less chance of minor bleeding problems. The blood salicylate level rises more slowly and lasts longer than with aspirin, therefore the drug does not have to be taken as often as aspirin.

Disalcid should be avoided in children during chicken pox or influenza because of the possibility of Reye syndrome.

Some doctors do not believe that the anti-inflammatory activity of Disalcid is as good as that of aspirin. Other doctors believe the effects are identical. It seems likely that Disalcid is less toxic than ordinary aspirin, but it is not clear that it is as effective a drug. It finds particular use in patients who have had problems with stomach upset from ordinary aspirin or who are in high-risk groups for gastrointestinal bleeding episodes.

SPECIAL HINTS

If you note ringing in the ears or a decrease in your hearing, decrease the dose of Disalcid; it is just a little bit too high for best results. Keep track of your Disalcid intake and always tell the doctor exactly how much you are taking.

ECOTRIN

325 mg, 500 mg tablet or caplet
See acetylsalicylic acid (aspirin)

TRILISATE (choline magnesium trisalicylate)

500 mg capsule-shaped, pale pink, scored tablet
750 mg capsule-shaped, white, scored, film-coated tablet
1,000 mg capsule-shaped, red, scored, film-coated tablet

PURPOSE

To relieve pain; to reduce inflammation.

INDICATIONS

For mild pain relief of cartilage degeneration and local conditions. Also an anti-inflammatory agent.

DOSAGE

For pain, one or two 500 mg tablets every 12 hours. For anti-inflammatory activity, two to three tablets every 12 hours. Each 750 mg Trilisate capsule is equivalent in salicylate content to 10 grains of aspirin (two normal-sized aspirin tablets). Occasionally higher doses may be needed. The maximum effect is reached in two hours for pain effects; one to three weeks are required for anti-inflammatory action to take full effect.

SIDE EFFECTS

Common effects include nausea, vomiting, ringing in the ears, and decreased hearing. Each of these is reversible within a few hours if the drug dosage is decreased. Allergic reactions are rare but may include development of nasal polyps and wheezing. With an overdose of salicylate there can be very heavy and rapid breathing, which can lead to unconsciousness and coma.

Other NSAIDs

Aspirin is a "nonsteroidal anti-inflammatory drug," or NSAID. That is, it is not a corticosteroid (like prednisone), but it is an anti-inflammatory agent because it reduces inflammation. Some of the disadvantages of aspirin have been noted above. In anti-inflammatory doses side effects such as nausea, vomiting, and ringing in the ears are common. Some people can't tolerate these side effects. Others, either ill-advised or not persistent, don't really try. In addition, aspirin somewhat inconveniently requires a number of tablets and regular attention to the medication schedule. So a class of "aspirin substitutes" has been developed. In common medical usage, aspirin is not grouped with these other NSAIDs, although it really should be. (In the over-the-counter market, "aspirin substitute" usually refers to acetaminophen [Tylenol], which is discussed below as a pain reliever; acetaminophen is not an anti-inflammatory drug.)

There is a huge market for NSAIDs. Nearly every major drug company has tried to invent one and has promoted heavily whatever has been developed.

Commonly Used NSAIDs

Arthrotec, Celebrex, Clinoril, Daypro, Feldene, Indocin, Lodine, Mobic, Motrin, Naprosyn, Orudis, Relafen, Vioxx, Voltaren

Available evidence indicates that different drugs work best for different individuals. These drugs come from several different chemical families and are not interchangeable. You may have to try several to find the best. The most frequently used medications in this category are discussed below in alphabetical order, according to brand name. The generic name is given in parentheses.

ADVIL (ibuprofen)

See Motrin and Ibuprofen Sold Over the Counter

ALEVE (naproxen)

See Naprosyn and Naproxen Sold Over the Counter

ARTHROTEC (diclofenac plus misoprostil)

Tablets with 50 or 75 mg diclofenac and 200 micrograms misoprostil

PURPOSE

To reduce inflammation; to reduce pain; to reduce gastrointestinal side effects.

INDICATIONS

For anti-inflammatory action and pain relief.

DOSAGE

50 mg/200 twice daily or three times daily; 75 mg/200 twice daily.

SIDE EFFECTS

Gastrointestinal side effects occur, with the most common being irritation of the stomach lining, nausea, indigestion, and heartburn. Additionally, diarrhea is quite common. Hospitalization for gastrointestinal bleeding occurs in about 0.5% of those taking full doses for one year. Further side effects are discussed under Voltaren.

This is a combination drug, in which misoprostil is included to preserve prostaglandin in the stomach lining and to decrease the chance of serious side effects. It decreases serious side effects from the diclofenac by about half. This is sufficient to make it a safer drug, but probably still not the safest. Unfortunately, the addition of misoprostil also increases the toxicity for diarrhea, and many individuals have diarrhea resulting from the drug. As a result, the relatively minor symptoms such as nausea and diarrhea are not reduced over other drugs, although the serious side effects are.

SPECIAL HINTS

For stomach upset, take the pills after meals and skip a dose or two if necessary. Diarrhea may last only for a short time and may be mild, or it may necessitate reduction in dose or even switching to another drug. Check with your doctor if the distress continues. Maximum therapeutic effect is achieved after one to two weeks of treatment and you should be able to see a major effect in the first week if Arthrotec is going to be a really good drug for you. Drugs likely to be of equal or lesser toxicity include low-dose aspirin, Tylenol, Disalcid, Trilisate, Lodine, Relafen, and the COX-1 sparing drugs.

CELEBREX (celecoxib)

100 mg tablet

PURPOSE

To reduce inflammation; to reduce pain; to reduce gastrointestinal side effects.

INDICATIONS

For anti-inflammatory action and pain relief.

DOSAGE

For osteoarthritis, 200 mg daily or 100 mg twice daily; for rheumatoid arthritis, 100–200 mg twice daily.

SIDE EFFECTS

Minor gastrointestinal side effects are quite common and include nausea, indigestion, heartburn, and diarrhea. Other side effects seen with other NSAIDs are also seen on occasion. This is a COX-1-sparing (selective COX-2 inhibitor) drug. It has been designed to give near maximal safety against serious gastrointestinal problems. Ulcers are very rarely seen and serious GI side effects are likely to be extremely rare.

SPECIAL HINTS

This drug has been described in the lay press as a "super aspirin." However, it is *not* more powerful than previously available drugs. It should be safer. It is a new drug and some side effects may not yet have been discovered. It may be more expensive than alternatives. It is probably not safer than Disalcid or Tylenol.

For stomach upset, take the pills after meals and skip a dose or two if necessary. Antacids may be used for gastrointestinal problems and may help. Check with your doctor if the distress continues. You should be able to see a major effect in the first week or so if Celebrex is going to be a really good drug for you.

CLINORIL (sulindac)

150 mg, 200 mg hexagon-shaped, bright yellow tablet

PURPOSE

To reduce inflammation; to reduce pain.

INDICATIONS

For anti-inflammatory action and pain relief.

DOSAGE

One 150 mg tablet twice a day. This drug also comes in a 200 mg tablet and dosage may be increased to 200 mg twice a day if needed. Maximum recommended dose is 400 mg a day.

SIDE EFFECTS

Gastrointestinal side effects, with irritation of the stomach lining, are the most common, and include nausea, indigestion, and heartburn. Stomach pain has been reported in 10% of subjects, and nausea, diarrhea, constipation, headache, and rash in 3 to 9%. Ringing in the ears, fluid retention, itching, and nervousness have been reported. Allergic reactions are rare. The manufacturer does not recommend the use of aspirin in combination with this drug since aspirin apparently decreases absorption from the intestine. Hospitalization for gastrointestinal bleeding occurs in about 1% of those taking full doses for one year.

SPECIAL HINTS

Sulindac has no particular advantages over the other anti-inflammatory agents described in this section, except that it may cause the minor kidney side effects less frequently and therefore is sometimes used for people with heart or kidney problems. It is of moderate toxicity.

For stomach upset, take the pills after meals; skip a dose or two if necessary. Check with your doctor if the distress continues. Maximum therapeutic effect is achieved after about three weeks of treatment, but you should be able to see a major effect in the first week if sulindac is going to be a really good drug for you.

DAYPRO (oxaprozin)

600 mg caplet

PURPOSE

To reduce inflammation; to reduce pain.

INDICATIONS

For anti-inflammatory action and pain relief in osteoarthritis and rheumatoid arthritis.

DOSAGE

The usual daily dose in rheumatoid arthritis or severe osteoarthritis is 1,200 mg (two 600 mg caplets) taken once daily. For patients of lower body weight or with milder disease, an initial dosage of one 600 mg caplet per day might be appropriate.

SIDE EFFECTS

Daypro can cause serious side effects, including stomach ulcers and intestinal bleeding. Most common side effects are dyspepsia and abdominal pain. As with other NSAIDs, serious side effects, such as gastrointestinal bleeding, may result in hospitalization or even fatal outcomes.

SPECIAL HINTS

Daypro is one of the newer nonsteroidal drugs. Its overall toxicity is probably about average. It has no particular advantages over other NSAIDs although some people respond well to it. It should not be taken by pregnant or nursing women. Its principal feature is that it needs to be taken only once a day, since it has a long half-life. This is a convenience feature but it does suggest caution in dosage, particularly if the patient is older or has other disease problems, since the drug might accumulate in the body. The maximum daily dose is 1,800 mg, but this is seldom used.

FELDENE (piroxicam)

10 mg dark red and blue capsule
20 mg dark red capsule

PURPOSE

To reduce inflammation; to reduce pain.

INDICATIONS

For anti-inflammatory activity and mild pain in rheumatoid arthritis, local conditions, and sometimes cartilage degeneration (osteoarthritis).

DOSAGE

One 20 mg tablet once daily. Do not exceed this dosage. This is a long-acting drug, and it need be taken only once daily.

SIDE EFFECTS

The drug has been consistently recognized as one of the more toxic NSAIDs. Gastrointestinal symptoms that involve irritation of the stomach lining occur, including nausea, indigestion, and heartburn. Allergic reactions, including skin rashes and asthma, are very rare. Peptic ulceration can occur, and hospitalization for gastrointestinal bleeding is seen in about 2% of those who take full doses for one year. Because Feldene is so long lasting, it may be unusually toxic for elderly people or for people with liver and kidney problems.

SPECIAL HINTS

Some seven to twelve days are required before the benefits of Feldene are apparent, and full benefits may not be clear for six weeks or more. Aspirin, except in low dose, should be avoided. Dosage recommendations and indications for use in children have not been established. Some patients with rheumatoid arthritis or osteoarthritis prefer Feldene, particularly because of the convenience of the once-a-day dosage.

INDOCIN (indomethacin)

25 mg, 50 mg blue and white capsule
75 mg blue and white, sustained-release capsule
50 mg blue suppository

PURPOSE

To reduce inflammation; to reduce pain.

INDICATIONS

For reduction of inflammation and for pain relief.

DOSAGE

One 25 mg capsule three to four times daily. For some patients, doses totaling as high as 150 mg (six capsules) may be required each day. Indocin is also available in 50 mg capsules. The 75 mg sustained-release form, needs to be taken only twice daily.

SIDE EFFECTS

Irritation of the stomach lining, including nausea, indigestion, and heartburn, occurs in a number of people. Allergic reactions (including skin rash and asthma) are very rare. A substantial problem, not present with other drugs of this class, is headache and a bit of a goofy feeling. Hospitalization for gastrointestinal bleeding is seen in about 2% of those on full doses for one year. Indocin is one of the more toxic NSAIDs.

SPECIAL HINTS

Many doctors find Indocin to be rather weak for treatment of rheumatoid arthritis. Maximum effect may take three weeks or so, but you should be able to tell within one week if it is going to be a major help. Some studies suggest that Indocin actually *increases* the rate of cartilage destruction in osteoarthritis of the hip. Usually it should not be the first NSAID tried.

Indocin, despite its potential toxicity, is often very effective in ankylosing spondylitis, Reiter's syndrome, and psoriatic arthritis. If you take it after meals you will have less stomach irritation, but some people do not absorb the drug very well. So for maximum effect you need to take it on an empty stomach, and for maximum comfort on a full stomach. Trial and error may be necessary to establish the best regimen for you. When some individuals take aspirin with Indocin, the Indocin is not absorbed from the intestine. Usually you will not want to take these two drugs together since you will get more irritation of the stomach lining but no more therapeutic effect. If this drug makes you feel mentally or emotionally fuzzy for more than the first few weeks, we think that is a good reason to discuss a change in medication with your doctor.

LODINE (etodolac)

200 mg capsule, light gray with one red band or dark gray with two narrow bands
300 mg capsule, light gray with two narrow red bands

PURPOSE

To reduce inflammation; to reduce pain.

INDICATIONS

For anti-inflammatory action and pain relief.

DOSAGE

For osteoarthritis, initially 800 to 1,200 mg per day in several doses. Do not exceed 1,200 mg per day. Lodine is not currently recommended for rheumatoid arthritis.

SIDE EFFECTS

This drug is generally well tolerated although, as with all of the nonsteroidal agents, it can result in bleeding from the stomach and other gastrointestinal problems. Some studies suggest there are fewer ulcers with this drug than with some other NSAIDs; thus, it is relatively safe.

SPECIAL HINTS

Lodine is one of the newer nonsteroidal drugs. More studies are needed to determine its usefulness when compared with other nonsteroidal anti-inflammatory drugs. It has been found less useful in rheumatoid arthritis than other drugs of this class. It does have some advantages with regard to gastrointestinal toxicity, and serious side effects are relatively rare.

MOBIC (meloxicam)

7.5 mg tablet

PURPOSE

To reduce inflammation; to reduce pain; to reduce serious gastrointestinal side effects.

INDICATIONS

For anti-inflammatory action and pain relief.

DOSAGE

One or two 7.5 mg tablets daily.

SIDE EFFECTS

This is a preferential COX-1-sparing drug. As such, it is likely to have fewer serious gastrointestinal reactions than other drugs. It does not spare COX-1 as effectively as Celebrex or Vioxx. In high doses (22.5 to 30 mg daily—not recommended) it appears to be as toxic as the typical NSAID. At recommended doses it appears to be one of the safest agents.

Relatively minor gastrointestinal side effects such as nausea, indigestion, and heartburn are reasonably common. Allergic reactions are rare and the drug is generally among the best tolerated.

SPECIAL HINTS

Mobic's principal advantage is that of relative safety, although how this safety compares with that of the other less toxic NSAIDs is not established. Considerable international experience suggests that it is moderately effective and comparatively well tolerated. It is a long-acting drug and needs to be taken only once daily. With side effects, reduce the dose or skip a few days. If symptoms persist, check with your doctor. As with other new selective COX-1-sparing drugs, there may be side effects which have not yet been well established. Aspirin, except in very low doses, should not be taken with Mobic. Maximum effect is achieved after about two weeks of treatment.

MOTRIN (ibuprofen)

300 mg round, white tablet
400 mg round, red-orange tablet
600 mg oval, peach tablet
800 mg capsule-shaped, apricot tablet

Motrin, Advil, and Rufen are the same drug, ibuprofen, produced by different companies. The over-the-counter brands contain smaller doses of ibuprofen (200 mg) and are available without a prescription (see next section).

PURPOSE

To reduce inflammation; to reduce pain.

INDICATIONS

For anti-inflammatory action and pain relief.

DOSAGE

One or two 400 mg tablets three times daily. Maximum daily recommended dosage is 2,400 mg, or six tablets.

SIDE EFFECTS

Motrin has fewer serious side effects than the other "older" NSAIDs. Gastrointestinal side effects, with irritation of the stomach lining, are the most common, and include nausea, indigestion, and heartburn. Allergic reactions are rare and the drug is generally well tolerated. A very few individuals have been observed with *aseptic meningitis,* apparently related to this drug. Here the person experiences a headache, fever, and stiff neck, and examination of the spinal fluid shows an increase in spinal fluid protein and white blood cells. The syndrome goes away when the drug is stopped but can come back if the drug is given again. Occasionally individuals may retain fluid with this medication. Hospitalization for gastrointestinal bleeding is needed in about 0.5% of those who take full doses of 2,400 mg per day or more for one year.

SPECIAL HINTS

Motrin is not consistently useful for the treatment of rheumatoid arthritis. Overall, many doctors feel that it is one of the weaker therapeutic agents in this group. If you are not getting enough relief, you may wish to discuss a change in medication with your doctor. Avoidance of aspirin (other than in low doses) while taking Motrin is advisable. Motrin is absorbed reasonably well even on a full stomach, so if you have problems with irritations of the stomach take the drug after an antacid or after a meal. Maximum effect is achieved after about three weeks of treatment, but if it is going to be a really good drug for you, you should be able to see a major effect in the first week.

Ibuprofen Sold Over the Counter

The Food and Drug Administration has approved the sale of ibuprofen without a prescription in a smaller, 200 mg tablet size. This historic ruling added a third minor analgesic to aspirin and acetaminophen, and now naproxen (Aleve) and ketoprofen (Orudis) are also available over the counter. The decision was made after a careful review of many studies indicating that ibuprofen was as effective as the two previously available drugs, and possibly less toxic than aspirin for relieving minor pain. Advil, Nuprin, and Motrin are the trade names for over-the-counter ibuprofen, and they are heavily advertised and heavily used. Ibuprofen is now also present in many different over-the-counter medications, including Midol. Remember, NSAIDs should be taken with caution whether prescription or nonprescription. Many serious gastrointestinal problems are seen even in people taking self-prescribed drugs.

What does this availability over the counter mean for the patient with arthritis? Relatively little. Many arthritis patients need at least 2,400 mg of ibuprofen per day, and twelve Advil tablets a day rather than four to six prescription Motrin is a bit of a nuisance. And it is hard to save money since the cost per milligram is about the same by prescription as over-the-counter. If you need anti-inflammatory doses of ibuprofen you should be seeing your doctor every so often anyway, so do not use the availability of the product over the counter as an excuse to stay away from the doctor. Also, many health insurance plans will not pay for medication unless it is purchased by prescription. Our recommendation remains that ibuprofen for arthritis be used on a prescription basis unless just an occasional tablet is required for pain. Similar advice holds for naproxen or ketoprofen.

NAPROSYN (naproxen)

250 mg round, light yellow tablet
375 mg capsule-shaped, peach tablet
500 mg capsule-shaped, light yellow tablet

PURPOSE

To reduce inflammation; to reduce pain.

INDICATIONS

For anti-inflammatory action and pain relief.

DOSAGE

One tablet two or three times a day. Maximum recommended dosage is 1,000 mg a day.

SIDE EFFECTS

Gastrointestinal side effects, with irritation of the stomach lining, are the most common, and include nausea, indigestion, and heartburn. Skin rash and other allergic problems are very rare. Fluid retention has been reported in a few individuals. Hospitalization for gastrointestinal bleeding is required in approximately 1% of patients taking full doses for one year, making it about average in toxicity.

SPECIAL HINTS

Naprosyn has an advantage over some drugs in this class by having a longer half-life. Each tablet lasts eight to twelve hours. Thus, you do not have to take as many tablets as with the other medicines in this group. Naprosyn is one of the most popular of the drugs of this class. Generic naproxen is now available, since the original naproxen patent has expired, and is much less expensive. Naproxen is believed by many rheumatologists to be more effective than most other NSAIDs.

In general, if you are taking Naprosyn you should avoid aspirin, since it interferes with Naprosyn in some individuals. An exception: Small doses of aspirin (40–80 mg per day) used to thin the blood and prevent heart attacks may be used with Naprosyn. If you notice fluid retention, reduce your salt and sodium intake and discuss a change in medication with your doctor. If you have stomach irritation, try taking the tablets on a full stomach or after antacids. Although absorption may be slightly decreased, you may be more comfortable overall.

Naproxen Sold Over the Counter

In 1993 the Food and Drug Administration (FDA) approved naproxen for nonprescription use in a smaller (200 mg) tablet size, adding a fourth over-the-counter pain reliever to the previously available acetaminophen, aspirin, and ibuprofen. Its longer half-life means that it only needs to be taken every 8 to 12 hours. You should not take more than three tablets in 24 hours (people over age 65 should not exceed two tablets) except on your doctor's recommendation. As with over-the-counter ibuprofen, we believe that most arthritis patients should be using prescription naproxen under a doctor's supervision.

NUPRIN (ibuprofen)

200 mg yellow tablet or caplet

See Motrin and Ibuprofen Sold Over the Counter

ORUDIS, ORUVAIL (ketoprofen)

25 mg dark green and red capsule
50 mg dark green and light green capsule
75 mg dark green and white capsule

PURPOSE

To reduce inflammation; to reduce pain.

INDICATIONS

For anti-inflammatory action and pain relief.

DOSAGE

Orudis comes in 25 mg, 50 mg, and 75 mg capsules. Recommended daily dose is 150 to 300 mg divided into three or four doses. Oruvail is a more recently introduced variant of Orudis,with a longer half-life.

SIDE EFFECTS

As with other drugs of this group, the most frequent side effects are gastrointestinal. Irritation of the stomach lining can cause nausea, heartburn, and indigestion. Occasionally individuals note fluid retention. Allergic reactions such as rash or asthma are very rare. Hospitalization for gastrointestinal bleeding occurs in over 1% of those taking full doses for one year, making it a bit worse than average in the frequency of serious toxicity.

SPECIAL HINTS

Chemically, Orudis is related to ibuprofen, naproxen, and fenoprofen. If you experience irritation of the stomach, decrease the dose or spread the tablets out throughout the day. Absorption will be slightly deceased if you take the drugs after meals or antacids, but greater comfort may result. Ketoprofen is useful in rheumatoid arthritis. It has found use in degenerative arthritis of the hip and for treatment of local conditions. Like other drugs of this group, ketoprofen will be the preferred drug for certain individuals. Orudis is now available over the counter. Since it appears to be more toxic than ibuprofen or naproxen, it should probably not be used as an OTC drug of first choice, and should be taken regularly only under a doctor's supervision.

RELAFEN (nabumetone)

500 mg oval, film-coated tablet
750 mg oval, film-coated tablet

PURPOSE

To reduce inflammation; to reduce pain.

INDICATIONS

For anti-inflammatory action and pain relief in patients with osteoarthritis and rheumatoid arthritis.

DOSAGE

Therapy is usually initiated at a dose of 1,000 mg daily, then adjusted, if needed, on the basis of clinical response.

SIDE EFFECTS

This is a relatively new drug, and it has been developed in part to minimize toxic effects on the stomach lining. It appears to be among the least toxic NSAIDs, with less than 0.5% serious gastrointestinal events each year. On the other hand, reductions in the frequency of major ulcers and of bleeding from the stomach have not yet been proved beyond doubt. Diarrhea is said to occur in 14% of people with this drug, heartburn in 13%, and abdominal pain in 12%. These figures are not very different from those of other NSAIDs.

SPECIAL HINTS

Do not exceed 2,000 mg per day. The lowest effective dose should be used if you are going to be taking this drug for a while. Many rheumatologists believe this to be a relatively weak NSAID.

VIOXX (rofecoxib)

12.5 mg tablet

PURPOSE

To reduce inflammation; to reduce pain.

INDICATIONS

For anti-inflammatory action and pain relief in rheumatoid arthritis and osteoarthritis.

DOSAGE

One or two tablets (12.5 mg to 25 mg) daily. This drug has a long half-life and needs to be taken only once daily.

SIDE EFFECTS

This is one of the new COX-1-sparing (COX-2 selective inhibitor) NSAIDs and has been designed to minimize serious gastrointestinal (GI) side effects—those that require hospitalization or are life threatening. Premarketing data suggest that it causes ulcers very rarely and that serious GI events are also very unusual. Thus, it appears to be one of the safest of the NSAIDs. Still, experience with it is limited, and there are some concerns about edema (swelling) and other relatively minor side effects. All of the usual NSAID problems with nausea, heartburn, dyspepsia, and diarrhea occur, although they are relatively infrequent. Allergic reactions are very rare.

SPECIAL HINTS

This appears to be a very safe drug. This and other selective COX-1-sparing drugs are believed to represent a major advance in safety. It is important to remember that Vioxx, as with the other new COX-1-sparing agents, is *not* more effective than older drugs; the advantage lies in the decrease in toxicity. Some data suggest that it might not always be quite as effective as some other NSAIDs. It is likely to be more expensive than the older drugs. You should be able to see an effect in one to two weeks if this drug is going to be a good one for you. Aspirin, except in low doses to prevent heart disease, should be avoided while taking Vioxx, since aspirin inhibits COX-1 and might increase Vioxx's toxicity.

VOLTAREN, CATAFLAM (diclofenac)

25 mg round, yellow, film-coated tablet
50 mg round, light brown, film-coated tablet
75 mg round, white, film-coated tablet

PURPOSE

To reduce inflammation; to reduce pain.

INDICATIONS

For anti-inflammatory action and pain relief.

DOSAGE

Usually one tablet (25 mg, 50 mg, or 75 mg) two or three times a day. The maximum recommended dosage is 200 mg per day.

SIDE EFFECTS

The most frequent side effects are gastrointestinal. As with other drugs of this group, irritation of the stomach lining can cause nausea, heartburn, and indigestion. Occasionally individuals may note fluid retention. Allergic reactions such as rash or asthma are very rare. Hospitalization for gastrointestinal bleeding probably occurs in about 1% of those taking full doses for one year, making it about average in risk for serious toxicity.

SPECIAL HINTS

Voltaren is the most frequently used nonsteroidal medication worldwide. The FDA was slow to review it, in part because of fear it would lead to more frequent liver problems. This does not appear to be a major problem, but periodic blood tests for liver toxicity are recommended by some.

Voltaren comes with an "enteric coating" designed to improve stomach tolerance; this is probably not effective. In case of irritation of the stomach, decrease the dose or spread the tablets out throughout the day. Absorption will be slightly decreased if you take the drug after meals or after antacids, but greater comfort may result.

Voltaren is useful in rheumatoid arthritis, degenerative arthritis, and treatment of local conditions. Certain individuals will prefer Voltaren to other drugs of this group. Cataflam is a derivative drug; its uses are in short-term pain relief and not arthritis treatment.

Less Frequently Used NSAIDs
Ansaid, Dolobid, Meclomen, Nalfon, Tolectin, Toradol

A number of NSAIDs have little advantage over alternatives and have gradually fallen into relative disuse. They may, however, have advantages for individual patients, so follow your doctor's advice. They are not discussed in detail here.

Ansaid (flurbiprofen) is an average NSAID that has had considerable use in Europe and moderate use in the United States. Its toxicity is about average, as is its effectiveness.

Dolobid (diflunisal) is an average NSAID without particular advantages. It causes more diarrhea than is average for drugs of this class.

Meclomen (meclofenemate) is probably the most toxic NSAID, taking all complications into account. It causes serious gastrointestinal effects more frequently than most other NSAIDs, and causes more frequent diarrhea than the other drugs. It is not recommended for children, and its effects have not been studied in patients with severe rheumatoid arthritis.

Nalfon (fenoprofen) was one of the earlier NSAIDs introduced. Its toxicity is relatively high and its effectiveness only average, so it has gradually declined in usage.

Tolectin (tolmetin sodium) has greater than average toxicity and seldom has benefit over alternative drugs. It needs to be taken three or four times daily since it has a fairly short half-life.

Toradol (ketorolac) is a drug used for short-term relief of pain, as in a postsurgical period. Toradol is not recommended for long-term use. It finds little use in arthritis except over periods of a week or less, and all of its side effects may not be known.

TYLENOL (acetaminophen)

325 mg white tablet or caplet
500 mg white tablet or caplet
500 mg yellow and red gel capsule

PURPOSE

To relieve pain.

INDICATIONS

Mild to moderate pain, particularly with cartilage degeneration (osteoarthritis) and in RA patients on DMARDs.

DOSAGE

Not to exceed 3,000 to 4,000 mg per day.

SIDE EFFECTS

Acetaminophen is the safest pain reliever currently known. It does not cause serious gastrointestinal bleeding, the most feared side effect of the NSAIDs. For most people it has no toxicity whatsoever. Unlike the NSAIDs, acetaminophen usually does not upset the stomach, does not cause ringing in the ears, does not affect the clotting of the blood, and does not interact with other medications. It is about as safe as can be. Nevertheless, nothing is perfect. Tylenol can be dangerous in overdose, and must be stored where children cannot reach it. When taken as an intentional overdose by adults—or as an accidental overdose in children—very severe liver reactions can result. These reactions can cause liver failure, need for liver transplant, or death. Liver reaction also occurs, though very rarely, when acetaminophen is taken in common with very large amounts of alcohol. Thus, recommended doses should never be exceeded, and heavy drinkers should avoid the drug or use it in no more than half doses. It has become fashionable for some to suggest that persons who drink any alcohol at all should avoid acetaminophen, but this is not accurate; moderate acetaminophen doses and moderate alcohol intake can coexist. Moreover, use of alcohol in high amounts theoretically increases the gastrointestinal toxicity of all of the NSAIDs, so alcohol moderation is just as important for those drugs. Acetaminophen may interact adversely with Coumadin, a blood-thinning drug. All in all, acetaminophen is the safest drug we have available for treatment of moderate to minor pain, but like all drugs, it should be treated with respect.

SPECIAL HINTS

Acetaminophen is a pain reliever with approximately the same power as most of the NSAIDs. However, it has no anti-inflammatory action at all. Hence, for a long time it was thought to have a very limited role in treatment of arthritis. Recent studies have shown, however, that for many people with osteoarthritis, Tylenol can be as effective as NSAIDs. In rheumatoid arthritis, Tylenol can be used to give pain relief while the major disease-modifying drugs (DMARDs), discussed below, are relied upon for the required anti-inflammatory activity. Tylenol is not a perfect pain reliever for everyone, but it is a drug that should be more frequently used by those for whom it is effective at relieving pain. It is relatively inexpensive.

Soon-to-be-released Nonsteroidal Medications

Some new NSAIDs, relatively similar to those just discussed, are in the process of review by the Food and Drug Administration. Many of these drugs are currently being used in other countries and appear to have a role in the treatment of arthritis. Judging from current knowledge, none of these new NSAIDs will be dramatically different from drugs already available. Also, a new drug is less well understood in terms of toxicity and benefits than a drug that has already been widely used. On the other hand, individual patients often do better with one or another nonsteroidal drug, so a wide choice of drugs is helpful for finding the drug that causes you the least toxicity and gives you the most benefit.

Some of these drugs have been formulated to have less gastrointestinal toxicity than their predecessors, and they may be safer. Sometimes, however, the agents that cause the fewest side effects turn out to be the least powerful drugs for the management of arthritis.

In general, when considering one of the new agents, rely on your doctor's advice. Acetaminophen (Tylenol) is among the safest of pain relievers. If you have been having a lot of trouble with stomach upset from drugs, then it might be a good idea to try one of the agents that causes less gastrointestinal difficulty, such as Disalcid, Trilisate, Relafen, Celebrex, or Vioxx. If you have not been getting the desired effect from the drugs of one chemical class, sometimes it is useful to try the drugs of a different class. It is possible that some new drugs will be better for rheumatoid arthritis and others better for osteoarthritis or other forms of arthritis. But treat each of these drugs with respect and consider that it is always possible for a drug, particularly a new drug, to be responsible for a new symptom that develops while you are taking the medication.

Corticosteroids

Over 50 years ago, a widely heralded miracle occurred: the introduction of cortisone for the treatment of rheumatoid arthritis. For people with rheumatoid arthritis and other forms of synovitis, the swelling and pain in their joints suddenly and dramatically decreased, as did the overall severity of their disease. They felt fine. The Nobel prize for medicine was awarded to the doctors who developed this drug.

The initial enthusiasm for cortisone in arthritis was tremendous. But slowly, over the following years, the cumulative side effects of cortisonelike drugs were recognized. For many individuals, the side effects were clearly greater than any benefits obtained. Cortisone became the model of a drug that provides early benefits but late penalties. Now, with a half century of experience with corticosteroids (also called corticoids or steroids), our perspective is more complete. They represent a major treatment for arthritis, but their use is appropriate in only a few cases, and then only with attention to potential complications. They appear effective in treating rheumatoid arthritis over a year or so, but over the long term they actually increase disability, mortality, and susceptibility to NSAID gastrointestinal side effects.

Steroids are natural hormones manufactured by the adrenal glands. When used medically, they are given in doses somewhat higher than the amounts the body generally makes. In these doses they suppress the function of your own adrenal glands and lead to a kind of drug dependency as the adrenal gland slowly shrinks from disuse. After many months of steroid use, the drug must be withdrawn slowly to allow your own adrenal gland to return to full function; otherwise an "adrenal crisis" can occur in which you just don't have enough hormone. Steroids must be taken exactly as directed, and a physician's close advice is always required.

Steroids used in treating arthritis are very different from the sex steroids, or androgens, taken by athletes and bodybuilders, often illegally. These other steroids have no role in treating arthritis and, indeed, shouldn't be used by athletes either.

The side effects of corticosteroids can be divided into categories based on the length of time you have been taking the steroid and the dose prescribed. If you have been taking steroids for less than one week, side effects are quite rare, even if the dose has been high.

If you have been taking high doses for one week to one month, you are at risk for development of ulcers, mental changes including psychosis or depression, infection with bacterial germs, or acne. The side effects of steroid treatment become most apparent after one month to one year of medium to high dosage. The individual becomes fat in the central parts of the body, with a buffalo hump on the lower neck and wasting of the muscles in the arms and legs. Hair growth increases over the face, skin bruises appear, and stretch marks develop over the abdomen. After years of steroid treatment (even with low doses) there is loss of calcium, resulting in fragile bones. Fractures can occur with only slight injury, particularly in the spine. Cataracts slowly develops and the skin becomes thin and translucent. Some physicians believe that hardening of the arteries occurs more rapidly and that there may be complications of inflammation of the arteries. Blood pressure may increase.

Many of these side effects will occur in everyone who takes sufficient doses of cortisone or its relatives for a sufficient period. The art of managing arthritis with corticosteroids involves knowing how to minimize these side effects. Your physician will work with you to keep the dose as low as possible at all times. If possible, you may be instructed to take the drug only once daily rather than several times daily, since there are fewer side effects when it is taken this way. If you are able to take the drug only every other day, this is even better, for the side effects are then quite minimal. Unfortunately, many people find that the dosage schedules that cause the fewest side effects also give them the least relief.

Steroids are always to be used with great respect and caution. The number of experienced doctors using low-dose corticosteroid treatment in a few patients with rheumatoid arthritis is increasing, but only slightly, demonstrating that the proper indications for use of these drugs are still somewhat controversial. High-dose cortisone treatment for uncomplicated rheumatoid arthritis has long been considered bad medical practice in the United States; it remains the essence of some quack treatments of arthritis, such as those available in Mexican border towns. Corticosteroids are harmful in infectious arthritis and should not be given by mouth in local conditions or in osteoarthritis.

There are three ways to give corticosteroids: by mouth, by vein, or by injection into the painful area. Prednisone is the steroid usually given by mouth and is the steroid discussed here. There are perhaps ten different steroid drugs now available. Prednisone, methylprednisolone, Decadron, and Aristocort are among the most commonly used. The fluorinated steroids, such as triamcinolone, cause greater problems with muscle wasting than does prednisone. The steroids sold by brand name are about 20 times as expensive as prednisone and do not have any major advantages. Hence, there is little reason to use any of these other compounds.

PREDNISONE

Dosages of 1 mg to 50 mg are available

PURPOSE

To reduce inflammation; to suppress immunological responses.

INDICATIONS

For suppression of serious systemic manifestations of connective-tissue disease, such as kidney involvement. In selected cases, low-dose use to suppress the inflammation of rheumatoid arthritis.

DOSAGE

The body normally makes the equivalent of about 5 to 7.5 mg of prednisone each day. "Low-dose" prednisone treatment is from 5 to 10 mg. A "moderate dose" ranges from 15 to 30 mg per day, and a "high dose" from 40 to 60 mg per day, or even higher. The drug is often most effective when given in several doses throughout the day, but side effects are least when the same total daily dose is given as infrequently as possible.

SIDE EFFECTS

Prednisone causes all of the corticosteroid side effects described above. Allergy is extremely rare. Side effects are related to dose and to duration of treatment. They can be major and can include fatal complications. Psychological dependency often occurs and complicates efforts to get off the drug once you have begun.

SPECIAL HINTS

Discuss the need for prednisone carefully with your doctor before beginning treatment. The decision to start steroid treatment for a chronic disease is a major one, and you want to be sure that the drug is essential. You may want a second opinion if the explanation does not completely satisfy you. When you take prednisone, follow your doctor's instructions closely. With some drugs it does not make much difference if you start and stop them on your own, but prednisone must be taken extremely regularly and exactly as prescribed. You will want to help your doctor decrease your dose of prednisone whenever possible, even if this does cause some increase in your symptoms.

A strange thing can happen when you reduce the dose of prednisone; a syndrome called *steroid fibrositis* can cause increased stiffness and pain for a week to ten days after each dose reduction. Sometimes this is wrongly interpreted as a return of the arthritis, and the reduction in dosage is unnecessarily stopped. If you are going to take prednisone for a long time, ask your doctor about taking some vitamin D along with it. There is some evidence that the loss of bone, the most critical long-term side effect, can be reduced if you take vitamin D (usually prescribed as 50,000 units once or twice a month) together with adequate calcium.

If you are having some side effects, ask your doctor about once-a-day or every-other-day use of the prednisone. Watch your salt and sodium intake and keep it low, since there is already a tendency to retain fluid with prednisone. Watch your diet as well, since you will be fighting a tendency to put on fat. If you stay active and limit the calories you take in, you can minimize many of the ugly side effects of the steroid medication and can improve the strength of the bones and the muscles. If you are taking a corticosteroid other than prednisone by mouth, ask your physician if it is all right to switch to the equivalent dose of prednisone.

STEROID INJECTIONS: Depo-medrol, other brands

PURPOSE

To reduce inflammation in a local area.

INDICATIONS

Noninfectious inflammation and pain in a particular region of the body. Or a widespread arthritis with one or two areas causing most of the problem.

DOSAGE

Dosage varies depending on the preparation and purpose. The frequency of injection is more important. Usually injections should be no more than every six weeks. Many physicians set a limit of three injections in a single area.

SIDE EFFECTS

Steroid injections resemble a very short course of prednisone by mouth and therefore have few side effects. They result in a high concentration of the steroid in the area that is inflamed and can have quite a pronounced effect in reducing this inflammation. If a single area is injected many times, the injection appears to cause damage in that area. This has resulted in serious problems in frequently injected areas, such as the elbows of baseball pitchers. Some studies suggest that as few as ten injections in the same place can cause increased bone destruction. Hence, most doctors stop injecting well before this time.

SPECIAL HINTS

If one area of your body is giving you a lot of trouble, an injection frequently makes sense. The response to the first injection will tell you quite accurately how much sense it makes. If you get excellent relief that lasts for many months, reinjection is indicated if the problem returns. The steroid injections contain a long-acting steroid, but it is in the body for only a few days. The effects may last much longer than this, however, since a cycle of inflammation and injury may be broken by the injection. If you get relief for only a few days, then injection is not going to be a very useful treatment for you. If you get no relief at all or an increase in pain, this is an obvious sign that other kinds of treatment should be sought. If you can find a "trigger point" on your body where pressure reproduces your major pain, then injection of this trigger point is frequently beneficial. Occasionally persons with osteoarthritis get benefit from injections, but injections usually are not helpful unless there is inflammation in the area.

CHAPTER 15

Disease-modifying Antirheumatic Drugs (DMARDs)

The anti-inflammatory drugs discussed in Chapter 14 are symptomatic medications only. They don't do anything basic to control arthritis over the long term. For rheumatoid arthritis and other forms of synovitis, there is a much more important class of drugs. Collectively, these drugs are usually called disease-modifying antirheumatic drugs, or DMARDs. They also have been called slow-acting antirheumatic drugs (SAARDs), or, inappropriately, remission-inducing drugs (RIDs). While they rarely induce true remission, in which the disease does not come back after the drug is stopped, they are much more effective anti-inflammatory agents than nonsteroidal anti-inflammatory drugs (NSAIDs), and a number of DMARDs have been conclusively shown to slow the process of joint destruction in rheumatoid arthritis. DMARDs are the most important drugs for rheumatoid arthritis and are often used in other inflammatory conditions.

A revolution in thinking about rheumatoid arthritis treatment is occurring. It used to be thought that DMARDs should be reserved for late use in patients with exceptionally severe disease of many years that could not be controlled with lesser agents. Now it is increasingly recognized that these drugs should be started early, and should be regarded as the backbone of treatment for rheumatoid arthritis. In general, patients with significant rheumatoid arthritis should be on one or another of these agents throughout the entire course of the disease. If you suspect rheumatoid arthritis, you should see a rheumatologist familiar with the use of DMARDs *as early as possible.*

This shift from considering DMARDs as powerful drugs to be kept in reserve to considering them front-line treatment came about because of a recognition of the serious complications of rheumatoid arthritis, the substantial side effects related to gastrointestinal bleeding from the NSAIDs, a reassuring safety profile for these stronger drugs, and the availability of a larger number of drugs of this class. In general, these drugs are about as safe as the moderate toxicity NSAIDs. Usually the good effects from these agents last only a few years, and so a strategy of using them sequentially, or even in combination, is required.

There are now 11 of these agents available, and more are under development. The 11 are intramuscular gold, oral gold, D-penicillamine, hydroxychloroquine, sulfasalazine, methotrexate, azathioprine, cyclosporine, leflunomide, etanercept, and infliximab. The last three are new and potentially quite exciting drugs. Methotrexate has become the most frequently used of these agents. Minocycline, also discussed below, may also be a DMARD, but this is not yet established. Cyclophosphamide (Cytoxan) is also a DMARD, but it is seldom used because of severe toxicity.

Gold (Intramuscular or Oral) and Penicillamine

These are major-league drugs, although no one knows exactly why they are so effective in so many individuals, and they are now used less frequently than the newer drugs. They provide dramatic benefits to over two-thirds of persons with severe rheumatoid arthritis. Each has major side effects that require stopping treatment in at least one-quarter of users and that may, in rare cases, be fatal. Gold salts and penicillamine are two very different kinds of drugs, but there are striking similarities in the types and magnitude of good effects and in the types of side effects. Neither appears to be of use in any disease other than rheumatoid arthritis, but the scientific proof of their effectiveness in rheumatoid arthritis is impressive.

These agents can result in complete remission of the arthritis, at least for the period while the drug is continued. In perhaps one-quarter of users the disease will actually be so well controlled that neither doctor nor patient can find any evidence of it. Usually these drugs have to be continued in order to maintain the remission. For reducing inflammation, the effects of these drugs can be more dramatic than with any other agents, except possibly methotrexate, leflunomide, or the anti-TNF drugs discussed below (see Cytokine Treatments). Individuals who use these drugs must accept certain significant hazards, but there is a good chance of major benefit. In rheumatoid arthritis, these drugs also have been shown to retard the process of joint destruction.

If you are not able to tolerate one of these drugs, you may be able to tolerate the other. After failure with one drug, the chances of success with the second drug decrease a little, but success is still common.

Which of these drugs should be used first? No one knows. In England penicillamine is usually used first. In the United States, it is gold. Gold requires a visit to the doctor every week for a while. The total cost of the initial course of injectable gold, including blood tests, may be $1,500 or more. Penicillamine can be taken by mouth, and while the drug itself is expensive, the total cost may be less. In terms of effectiveness and risk, you can consider these two drugs about the same. Both are sound drugs but have been largely superseded by newer drugs, particularly methotrexate.

MYOCHRISINE, SOLGANOL (gold salts)

PURPOSE

To reduce inflammation and retard disease progression.

INDICATIONS

Rheumatoid arthritis and some other forms of synovitis.

DOSAGE

50 mg per week by intramuscular injection for 20 weeks, then one to two injections per month thereafter. Many doctors use smaller doses for the first two injections to test for allergic reactions. Sometimes doctors will give more or less than this standard dosage depending upon your body size and response to treatment. "Maintenance" gold treatment refers to injections after the first 20 weeks (which result in a total of about 1,000 mg of gold). The dosage and duration of maintenance therapy vary quite a bit; with good responses the gold maintenance may be continued for many years, with injections given every two to four weeks.

SIDE EFFECTS

The gold salts accumulate very slowly in the tissues of the joints and in other parts of the body. Hence, side effects usually occur only after a considerable amount of gold has been received, although allergic reactions can occur even with the initial injection. The major side effects have to do with the skin, kidneys, and blood cells. The skin may develop a rash, usually occurring after ten or more injections, with big red spots or blotches, often itchy. If the rash remains a minor problem, the drug may be cautiously continued, but occasionally a very serious rash occurs following gold injections.

The kidney can be damaged so that protein leaks out of the body through the urine. This is called *nephrosis* or the *nephrotic syndrome* if it is severe. When it is recognized and the drug is stopped, the nephrosis usually goes away, but cases have been reported in which it did not reverse. The blood cell problems are the most dangerous. They can affect either the white blood cells or the platelets, those blood cells that control the clotting of the blood. In each case, the gold causes the bone marrow to stop making the particular blood cell. If the white cells are not made, the body becomes susceptible to serious infections. If the platelets are not made, the body is subject to serious bleeding episodes that can be fatal. These problems almost always reverse when the drug is stopped, but reversal may take a number of weeks, during which time the person is at risk for a major medical problem.

There are other side effects, such as ulcers in the mouth, a mild toxic effect on the liver, or nausea, but they usually are not as troublesome as the side effects just described. Overall, about one-quarter of users have to stop their course of treatment because of side effects. One or two percent of users experience a potentially serious side effect; other side effects don't really cause much of a problem. Less than one time in a thousand there may be a fatal side effect. With careful monitoring, the drug is reasonably safe and its benefits justify its use, since over 70% of those treated with gold show moderate or marked improvement. However, you must maintain your respect for this treatment and keep up regular blood tests to detect early side effects. One final note: Most side effects occur during the initial period of 20 injections. Serious side effects during the maintenance period are less common.

SPECIAL HINTS

You must be patient with gold treatment. The gold accumulates slowly in the body and good responses are almost never seen in the first ten weeks of treatment. Improvement begins slowly after that, and major improvement is usually evident by the end of 1,000 mg, or 20 weeks. Similarly, if the drug is stopped, it requires many months before the effect is totally lost. In one famous study, the gold group was still doing better than the control group two years after the drug had been stopped, although most of the effect of the drug had been lost by that time. After a side effect has been dealt with or has subsided, many doctors will suggest that the drug be tried again. Often this can be worthwhile if the approach is very cautious, since the drug is frequently tolerated the second time around. At our Arthritis Center we do not try gold salts again if there has been a problem with the blood, but we may use it again, cautiously, after mild skin reactions or mild amounts of protein loss through the urine.

To minimize the chance of serious side effects, most doctors recommend checking the urine for protein leakage, checking the white cells and the platelets, and asking the patient about skin rash before every injection. This is good practice. Unfortunately, the combination of 20 doctor visits, 20 injections, 20 urinalyses, 20 blood counts, and so forth, makes the cost of initiating gold treatment approximately $1,500. There are some ways to decrease this cost while preserving safety. You can ask your doctor to prescribe some test kits so that you can test your urine for protein at home. This is a very easy technique. You can ask if it is possible to have just a platelet smear and a white count rather than a complete blood count each time. You can inquire whether it is possible to have the nurse give an injection after checking the blood count without actually having a doctor visit every week. And some people have successfully been giving themselves their own shots at home with the help of a family member, although many doctors consider this unacceptable.

RIDAURA (auranofin)

3 mg brown and white capsule with tapered ends

PURPOSE

To reduce inflammation in rheumatoid arthritis and retard disease progression. (This drug is "oral gold.")

INDICATIONS

For anti-inflammatory activity in rheumatoid arthritis.

DOSAGE

Average dosage is 6 mg daily. The drug is slowly absorbed and distributed through the body, and weeks to months may be required before full therapeutic effect is achieved.

SIDE EFFECTS

The most common side effect is dose-related diarrhea, which occurs at some time in approximately one-third of treated patients and requires discontinuation in 10 to 20% of patients. Skin rash has occurred in 4%, mild kidney problems in 1%, and problems with the platelets in 0.5% of patients.

SPECIAL HINTS

Ridaura is a helpful drug for some rheumatoid arthritis patients, but it is seldom helpful unless it is the first DMARD selected. It is not effective in osteoarthritis, gout, or minor rheumatic conditions. It may or may not have an eventual role in psoriatic arthritis, ankylosing spondylitis, and the arthritis of children. It is not nearly as strong a DMARD as intramuscular gold. If diarrhea is encountered, the dose should be reduced. As with intramuscular gold injections, patients should be monitored periodically for blood complications, skin rash, and protein loss in the urine. Follow your doctor's advice for the particular tests required and the frequency with which they are needed. Ridaura is most useful in the first year or so of rheumatoid arthritis.

PENICILLAMINE (cuprimine)

125 mg gray and yellow capsule
250 mg yellow capsule

PURPOSE

To reduce inflammation and retard disease progression.

INDICATIONS

Rheumatoid arthritis and some other forms of synovitis.

DOSAGE

Usually 250 mg (one 250 mg tablet, or two 125 mg tablets) per day for one month, then two tablets (500 mg) a day for one month, then three tablets (750 mg) per day for one month, and finally four tablets (1,000 mg) per day. Dosage usually is increased slowly, and may be increased even more slowly than this. After a positive response, the drug can be continued indefinitely, sometimes at a reduced dosage. If a good result is obtained earlier, the patient can stop with the lower dose.

SIDE EFFECTS

Side effects closely parallel those noted above for gold injections. The major side effects are skin rash, protein leakage through the urine, or a decrease in production of the blood cells. Additionally, individuals may have nausea, or may notice a metallic taste in the mouth or a decreased sense of taste.

Penicillamine weakens the connective tissue so that the healing of a cut is delayed, and a scar may not have the same strength it would have without the penicillamine. Stitches following a cut should be left in for a longer period, and surgery under these circumstances may be more difficult.

SPECIAL HINTS

Penicillamine takes a number of months to reach its full therapeutic effect and the effect persists for a long time after you stop taking the drug. Responses usually take from three to six months but can be as late as nine months after the drug is begun. Because of the risk of side effects, doctors have now adopted the "go low, go slow" approach given in the dosage schedule above. In the past, when full doses were begun earlier, the frequency of side effects was higher. Even now only about three-quarters of individuals will complete the treatment; the remainder will have some side effects—approximately the same as those listed for gold salts. The drug may be tried again after a mild side effect. We do not try the drug again if there has been a problem with the blood counts, but we may cautiously try it if there has been a minor problem with protein in the urine, a minor skin rash, or minor nausea.

Monitoring for side effects has to be carefully performed. Usually a blood count or smear, a urinalysis to test for protein leakage, and questioning of the person about side effects are required every two weeks or even more frequently. It should be noted that, with both penicillamine and gold, careful monitoring improves your chances of not having a serious side effect but does not eliminate the possibility. As with gold treatment, you can negotiate to have some of the drug monitoring done by a local laboratory and review the results yourself, check your own urine for protein, and so forth, if you desire. Most doctors who use these drugs a good deal have evolved some method of minimizing the cost of the monitoring. After the first six months side effects are relatively rare but still do occur. Some individuals will have an excellent response to the penicillamine even though they never get up to the full dosage of 1,000 mg per day.

Antimalarial and Antibiotic Medications

PLAQUENIL (hydroxychloroquine)

200 mg round, white, scored tablet

PURPOSE

To reduce inflammation and to retard disease progression in rheumatoid arthritis; to reduce disease activity in systemic lupus erythematosus (lupus).

INDICATIONS

Rheumatoid arthritis and systemic lupus erythematosus.

DOSAGE

One to two tablets (200 to 400 mg) per day.

SIDE EFFECTS

This is one of the best tolerated of all drugs used for rheumatoid arthritis, and side effects are unusual. With a very few people, gastric upset or muscular weakness may result. Consideration needs to be given to the possibility of retinal (eye) toxicity, which is an occasional complication of antimalarial drugs. This rare complication appears to be always reversible if the patient is regularly monitored by periodic eye examinations after the first year of treatment. The eye examination will detect any problems well before you notice any change in vision.

SPECIAL HINTS

Plaquenil takes six weeks to begin to show an effect, and full effect can take up to 12 weeks, so plan on at least a 12-month trial. The eye complications appear to be much less common with Plaquenil than with chloroquine, the earlier antimalarial drug. They are seldom, if ever, seen with less than one year of treatment at recommended dosage. Bright sunlight seems to increase the frequency of eye damage, so we recommend using sunglasses and wide-brimmed hats for sun protection. We recommend eye examinations after one year of continuous treatment and at 12-month intervals thereafter. This should give ample warning of any problems. Do not exceed two tablets daily. Since the drug is so well tolerated, both tablets may be taken together in the morning. The good effects of this drug are long-lasting and continue for weeks or months after the drug is stopped. Overall, this is one of the safest drugs available for treatment of rheumatoid arthritis and lupus; it should be used with respect but not fear.

AZULFIDINE (sulphasalazine)

Azulfidine EN-tabs: 500 mg orange, film-coated tablet

PURPOSE

To reduce inflammation and to retard disease progression in rheumatoid arthritis.

INDICATIONS

Rheumatoid arthritis and some other forms of synovitis.

DOSAGE

Three or four 500 mg tablets daily, taken in two or three doses. Dosage may be increased to as many as six 500 mg tablets, usually taken as two tablets three times daily.

SIDE EFFECTS

This is a sulfa drug and should not be taken by people with an allergy to sulfa, which is present in many antibiotics such as Septra and Gantrisin. Allergy is unusual, but may take the form of a rash, wheezing, itching, fever, or jaundice. Azulfidine may cause gastric distress or other side effects in some patients. Blood tests should be done every so often to detect any effects on the blood cells or platelets; such effects are rare. Most people, probably four out of five, experience no trouble whatsoever.

SPECIAL HINTS

Azulfidine is used in patients with inflammatory problems with the bowels, where it reduces the inflammation, at least in part because of an antibiotic effect on the bacteria that live in the bowel. British scientists have documented that it has a major effect on rheumatoid arthritis, and this has been confirmed by investigators in the United States. While it is an antibiotic, no one knows for sure how it works. But it is very effective in some patients. It takes a month or more before the effects begin to be noticed, and full effects may take three or more months. Usually if you are not going to tolerate the drug, you will know in a week or so.

MINOCIN (minocycline)

100 mg capsule

PURPOSE

To reduce inflammation in rheumatoid arthritis.

INDICATIONS

This drug was developed primarily as an antibiotic and has been in use for a long time. In rheumatoid arthritis it has proved effective with mild to moderate disease and is a good drug to try earlier in the course of the disease. Some doctors think it works in rheumatoid arthritis through its antibiotic actions, but others point out that it has profound chemical effects on the joint tissues as well. Its role in osteoarthritis is under investigation.

DOSAGE

200 mg (one 100 mg capsule twice a day).

SIDE EFFECTS

Minocycline is generally well tolerated. Be careful with sun exposure. In some people it can cause severe sunburn reactions. As a broad spectrum antibiotic it decreases the number of bacteria in the bowel. This can lead to overgrowth of other bacteria and resulting diarrhea. All of this happens surprisingly rarely. More commonly there can be overgrowth of a fungus, causing severe itching around the anus or white patches in the throat and esophagus. This is a signal to discontinue the drug and sometimes to take medication for the fungus infection. Rarely, some nausea and allergic reactions occur. A few patients have developed a lupuslike illness.

SPECIAL HINTS

In rheumatoid arthritis it can take several weeks to see the benefit. This drug is theoretically considered a DMARD, but it has not been shown to delay the progression of rheumatoid arthritis. It can be used in combination with any of the other DMARDs. Because it is not a very powerful anti-inflammatory drug, it should not be used as the sole drug over a long period unless the results are quite dramatic. Usually patients with rheumatoid arthritis will have to move on from minocycline to stronger drugs. Minocycline is inexpensive. It should not be used in children because of the chance of mottling of the developing teeth.

Immunosuppressant Drugs

Immunosuppressant drugs are very important DMARD agents for the management of rheumatoid arthritis. They are prescribed in rheumatoid arthritis because they can reduce the number of inflammatory cells present around the joint. They are very powerful and useful drugs. There are several exciting new drugs in this general category.

The immune response helps the body recognize and fight foreign particles and viruses. When it goes wrong, it can cause autoimmune disease. Antibodies from the immune system can attack the body's own tissues, causing disease. Immunosuppressant drugs can tone down this reaction.

Some of these drugs work by *cytotoxic* action. They kill rapidly dividing cells much like an X-ray beam. Since in some diseases the most rapidly dividing cells are the bad ones, the overall effect of the drugs is good. Others of these drugs antagonize a chemical system inside the cell, such as the purine system or the folate system. From the patient's standpoint, it doesn't really make much difference how the different drugs work.

A major short-term worry with many of these drugs is that they can destroy bone marrow cells. The bone marrow cells make red cells that carry oxygen, white cells that fight infection, and platelets that stop bleeding. Any of these blood cell types can be suppressed if you take enough immunosuppressant drugs.

Even if there seem to be enough white cells, infections can occur. These infections are often called "opportunistic," which means that they are caused by different kinds of germs than those that cause infections in healthy people. For example, patients with suppressed immune systems are often afflicted with herpes zoster (shingles), and can be prone to infections from types of fungi that are around all the time but seldom cause disease. Or a rare bacterial infection can occur. These infections can be difficult to treat and sometimes hard to diagnose.

For patients who have taken immunosuppressant drugs for several years, there is some concern about an increased risk of cancer. If such cancer happens at all, it appears to be quite rare. Present evidence suggests that leukemia can occasionally be caused by cytotoxic drugs such as cyclophosphamide, but not by methotrexate or azathioprine. Cyclophosphamide is now very rarely used in rheumatoid arthritis because of its toxicity.

Although there is some potential danger with these drugs, they actually may be no more dangerous than some of the drugs with which we have become more comfortable. The benefits can be enormous, and these drugs represent a tremendous advance in treatment of rheumatoid arthritis.

METHOTREXATE

2.5 mg round yellow tablet

PURPOSE

For reduction of inflammation and to retard disease progression.

INDICATIONS

Rheumatoid arthritis, dermatomyositis or polymyositis, psoriatic arthritis, other forms of synovitis.

DOSAGE

If taken orally, as is usual in rheumatoid arthritis, the dose is usually 5 to 20 mg per week given in two or three doses, twelve hours apart, sometimes as a single weekly dose. It should *not* be taken every day. It can be given as an injection as well, in which case doses may sometimes be as high as 40 or 50 mg per week (only when recommended by your doctor).

SIDE EFFECTS

These include opportunistic infections, mouth ulcers, and stomach problems. Damage to the liver, a special side effect of this drug, is particularly a problem if the drug is taken orally every day. When taken by mouth, this drug is absorbed by the intestine and passes through the liver on the way to general circulation. As a result, most doctors have discontinued this daily method of administration. Instead the drug is given intermittently, once a week, so that the liver has an opportunity to heal. Problems can still occur with the newer dose schedules, but are much less frequent. A severe problem with the lungs is occasionally seen with methotrexate. There remains uncertainty about whether lymphoma can very rarely occur.

Methotrexate can, in rare cases, damage the liver. Enzymes can leak out of damaged liver cells and this can be measured in the blood. Liver function tests are used to detect damage before it becomes severe. The tests include bilirubin (jaundice), serum albumin, and serum alkaline phosphatase. The most important, however, are the liver enzymes SGOT (also called AST or ASAT) and SGPT (also called ALT or ALAT). Usually test values should be below 40. With methotrexate therapy, enzyme levels are usually checked every four to eight weeks, at least for the first one or two years, and then, if results are normal, perhaps less often. If they are abnormal more than half of the time, it can be a signal to reduce the dose, stop the drug, or to consider a liver biopsy to see if any damage has occurred.

SPECIAL HINTS

This drug is extremely effective in many cases of rheumatoid arthritis and has become the preferred drug for many patients. Because of its remarkable effectiveness it is now the most frequently used of the DMARDs. Regular blood tests are required, as with all of these drugs. Some doctors recommend liver biopsy to be sure that the liver is normal before starting the drug. However, this procedure has some hazard and is not necessary as long as blood liver tests are normal before the drug is started. Since alcohol also can damage the liver, alcohol intake should be extremely moderate during methotrexate treatment. Some doctors recommend liver biopsy after a few years of treatment to make sure that no liver scarring has occurred. Current belief is that this is not necessary unless the liver blood tests are consistently abnormal. At this time there seem to be worse complications from liver biopsies (the death rate is between 1 in 1,000 and 1 in 10,000) than from methotrexate liver disease (only about 40 serious events reported). Patients who are taking Plaquenil together with methotrexate seem to have fewer liver test abnormalities. Some doctors like to prescribe folic acid along with methotrexate; this may help to reduce side effects.

IMURAN (azathioprine), 6-MP (6-mercaptopurine)

50 mg hourglass-shaped, yellow to off-white, scored tablet

PURPOSE

For immunosuppression.

INDICATIONS

Severe systemic lupus erythematosus (lupus), rheumatoid arthritis, psoriatic arthritis, steroid-resistant polymyositis or dermatomyositis.

DOSAGE

100 to 150 mg (two or three tablets) daily.

SIDE EFFECTS

Azathioprine (Imuran) and 6-mercaptopurine (6-MP) are closely related drugs with almost identical actions. Azathioprine is the more frequently used. Side effects include opportunistic infections and the possibility of cancer development after extended use. So far both effects are rare to absent in humans. Gastrointestinal (stomach) distress is occasionally noted. Hair loss is unusual, and there appears to be little effect on the sperm or the eggs. There are no bladder problems as with cyclophosphamide. Although liver damage has been reported, the drug is usually well tolerated.

SPECIAL HINTS

Regular blood tests are required. Patients taking Imuran or 6-MP should never take allopurinol (Zyloprim), a drug used to treat gout, at the same time since the combination of drugs can be fatal.

Once the patient responds to Imuran or 6-MP it is often possible to reduce the dose. Theoretically, this decreases the risk of late side effects.

Azathioprine has been shown to slow down the progression of rheumatoid arthritis and is very effective in some patients. Most people seem not to have any side effects, but there is still concern about what might happen over the long run.

ARAVA (leflunomide)

10, 20, or 100 mg tablet

PURPOSE

To reduce inflammation and to retard disease progression in rheumatoid arthritis.

INDICATIONS

For reduction of inflammation in moderate to severe rheumatoid arthritis.

DOSAGE

A loading dose of 100 mg is taken for three days, and then 20 mg per day after that. The standard maintenance dose is from 10 to 20 mg per day.

SIDE EFFECTS

Because this drug is new, some side effects may not have been recognized and long-term side effects are not known. The most frequent problems are skin rash, abdominal pain, diarrhea, and nausea. Occasionally there can be elevations of the liver enzymes or hair loss. Liver function tests are recommended at intervals of six to twelve weeks, at least for the first year or two of treatment.

SPECIAL HINTS

Leflunomide has been proven to modify the course of rheumatoid arthritis. While a new drug, its effectiveness appears to be quite similar to that of methotrexate, making it potentially a new advance and providing an important new alternative treatment for rheumatoid arthritis. It is chemically not related to other DMARDs. It appears that its action may be similar to that of Imuran, but it may be more predictably effective in rheumatoid arthritis. It may find a role in combination treatment with methotrexate or other DMARDs, although studies of such usage are not yet complete. It should not be taken by people with liver disease or with immune deficiency syndromes. It is not indicated for women who may become pregnant since the drug may persist for up to two years in the body. It has not been tested for safety and effectiveness in children. To minimize any risk of birth defects, men who wish to father a child should first stop the drug. A drug (cholestyramine) can be used to remove Arava from the body, and this can be accomplished in about two weeks. Arava appears to work by inhibiting pyrimidine synthesis, causing rapidly multiplying cells, such as inflammatory cells, to divide more slowly. Treatment effects are generally seen in the first month and reach their peak after three to six months.

SANDIMMUNE (cyclosporine)

25 mg capsule
100 mg capsule

PURPOSE

To reduce inflammation and disease progression in rheumatoid arthritis.

INDICATIONS

For reduction of inflammation in difficult, severe rheumatoid arthritis not responsive to other agents (not an approved use by the Food and Drug Administration).

DOSAGE

Use in rheumatoid arthritis is generally 3 to 5 mg per kilogram of body weight per day. For a 150-pound (70-kg) person, this is 200 to 350 mg per day.

SIDE EFFECTS

The principal adverse reactions are kidney failure, tremor, excess hair growth, and problems with the gums. In rheumatoid arthritis the major problem has been with the kidneys, and this sometimes requires discontinuation of the drug. The kidney failure is usually reversible.

SPECIAL HINTS

Cyclosporine was developed as a drug to prevent rejection of kidney, heart, and other organ transplants. It is a strong immunosuppressant. In rheumatoid arthritis its use is reserved for severely affected persons and it should be given only by physicians who are thoroughly familiar with its use. It can be very effective in some patients. The problem for rheumatoid arthritis patients is the kidney damage, which occurs at lower doses than in transplant patients. Hence, the dose must be kept lower. Some patients have had severe disease flare-ups after stopping cyclosporine. Researchers are exploring several ways to reduce the kidney problems, and there may be some progress in this area soon.

Cytokine Treatments

Cytokines are natural chemical substances that deliver important messages from cell to cell in the body. These messages often help in the regulation of chronic inflammation and tissue damage.

ENBREL (etanercept)

PURPOSE

For control of inflammation and to retard the progression of moderate to severe rheumatoid arthritis not completely responsive to other drugs.

DOSAGE

The standard dose is 25 mg given twice weekly by subcutaneous injection. Most patients quickly learn to perform the injections, although the first dose should be supervised by a health care professional.

SIDE EFFECTS

About one-third of patients develop minor injection site reactions. Severe infections can result, although these do not appear to be very frequent. There is some concern about possible development of lymphoma or other cancers, but to date there has been no suggestion of this. Allergic reactions, sometimes severe, can occur but appear to be very rare. In general, the drug is considered to be quite well tolerated.

SPECIAL HINTS

This is an extremely powerful and often dramatic drug for treatment of rheumatoid arthritis, even after other drugs have failed to completely control the disease. It appears to be effective in children with arthritis as well. It works by blocking the receptor for TNF-alpha, a cytokine. Some patients develop antibodies to their own tissues while taking the drug, but this is not seen today to be a major problem. A year of treatment costs approximately $12,000, making this the most expensive treatment for rheumatoid arthritis. Nevertheless, the often dramatic results may make this a good value for patients with very serious rheumatoid arthritis for whom other DMARDs have failed. Long-term side effects and effectiveness have not yet been determined.

REMICADE (infliximab)

PURPOSE

For treatment of severe rheumatoid arthritis not adequately controlled by other DMARD medications, generally taken together with methotrexate. For treatment of severe Crohn's disease of the bowel.

DOSAGE

Usual dose is 3 mg per kilogram of body weight, given by intravenous injection under medical supervision, at two-month intervals.

SIDE EFFECTS

Minor adverse events including headache, diarrhea, rash, and others are common but are generally well tolerated. There may be an increase in the rate of infections. There are theoretical concerns about development of lymphomas or other cancers but it is not yet known if these occur. Usually it is quite well tolerated.

SPECIAL HINTS

This very powerful new drug is an antibody to tumor necrosis factor (TNF), a cytokine. It is very effective in the treatment of Crohn's disease. Almost all of the studies for treatment of rheumatoid arthritis have been in combination with methotrexate, and when Remicade is added to methotrexate further dramatic improvement usually occurs. Improvement is usually seen after the first infusion but may continue after several more. Antibodies to DNA have occurred and there have been a small number of cases with a reversible condition similar to lupus. Long-term side effects and effectiveness against rheumatoid arthritis have not yet been established. Remicade treatment is expensive, with the cost of a year of treatment exceeeding $5,000. Nevertheless, this dramatic new treatment may have substantial value for patients with severe rheumatoid arthritis not adequately controlled by other DMARDs.

KINERET (anakinra)

PURPOSE

For control of inflammation and to retard the progression of severe rheumatoid arthritis not completely responsive to other DMARD medications.

INDICATIONS

Moderate to severe rheumatoid arthritis. May be used alone or in combination with other DMARDs except Enbrel or Remicade.

DOSAGE

The usual dose is 100 mg per day given by subcutaneous injection under medical supervision, generally at intervals of one to three months.

SIDE EFFECTS

Serious infections can occur in about 1–2% of patients. Decreased white cell counts can occur. Injection site reactions occur in most persons, but are usually mild and are uncommon after 4 weeks of treatment. Infections are most common when Enbrel and Kineret are used together and this combination should be used with great caution. Allergic and other types of side effects can occur. In general it is considered to be well-tolerated.

SPECIAL HINTS

This is a powerful new drug approved by the FDA in December 2001, although perhaps not quite as powerful as Remicade. It is a receptor antagonist for interleukin-1, a cytokine which increases inflammation, and is technically called "IL1ra". It has a distinct way of working, and might be effective when other cytokine treatments are not. It works well with methotrexate and other traditional DMARDs. Like other cytokine treatments it is expensive and cannot be taken by mouth.

CHAPTER 16

Painkillers and Other Approaches

This section is included mainly to emphasize that pain-reducing drugs, except plain acetaminophen (Tylenol), have little place in the treatment of arthritis. Tylenol, described in Chapter 14, is an important antiarthritis drug.

Consider the four major disadvantages of the strong painkillers. First, they don't do anything for the arthritis; they just cover it up. Second, they suppress the pain mechanism that tells you when you are doing something that is injuring your body. If you suppress the pain mechanism, you may injure your body without being aware of it. Third, the body adjusts to pain medicines, so that they aren't as effective over the longer term. This phenomenon is called *tolerance* and develops to some extent with all painkillers. Fourth, pain medicines can have major side effects. The side effects range from stomach distress to constipation to mental changes. Most of these drugs are "downers," which you don't need if you have arthritis. You need to be able to cope with a somewhat more difficult living situation than the average person. These drugs decrease your ability to solve problems.

Many individuals develop dependence on these agents. In arthritis, the addiction is somewhat different from what we usually imagine. Most people with arthritis are not truly physically addicted to codeine or Percodan or Demerol. They are psychologically dependent on these drugs as a crutch and become inordinately concerned with the attempt to eliminate every last symptom. These agents can conflict with the attempt to achieve independent living.

By and large, use these drugs only for the short term and only when resting the sore part, so that you don't reinjure it while the pain is suppressed. Drugs mentioned first in this list are less harmful than those listed later. Drugs to reduce inflammation, discussed in Chapter 14, may reduce pain through direct pain action as well as through reduction of inflammation. In osteoarthritis, plain acetaminophen (Tylenol, other brands) is often very useful as a nontoxic pain reliever and has become an increasingly useful drug.

The principles in the preceding paragraphs regarding the use and misuse of pain relievers hold for a number of less common pain relievers not described in the following section.

Drugs to Reduce Pain

DARVON (Darvon compound, Darvotran, Darvocet, Darvocet-N, propoxyphene)

Darvon: 32 mg, 65 mg pink capsule
Darvon compound: 32 mg gray and pink capsule; 65 mg gray and red capsule
Darvocet-N: 50 mg, 100 mg capsule-shaped, dark orange, coated tablet

PURPOSE

Pain relief.

INDICATIONS

For short-term use to decrease mild pain.

DOSAGE

One-half grain (32 mg) or 1 grain (65 mg) every four hours as needed for pain.

SIDE EFFECTS

These drugs have been widely used with a reasonably good safety record. In some cases side effects may be due to use of aspirin or other medication in combination with the Darvon. Most worrisome to us has been the mentally dull feeling that many individuals report, sometimes described as a gray, semi-unhappy fog. Others do not seem to notice this effect. Side reactions include dizziness, headache, sedation, paradoxical excitement, skin rash, and gastrointestinal disturbances.

SPECIAL HINTS

Darvon is not anti-inflammatory. The pain relief given is approximately equal to that of aspirin or acetaminophen in most cases. The drug is more expensive than aspirin or acetaminophen. It can induce dependence, particularly after long-term use.

CODEINE (Empirin #3, 4; Tylenol #1, 2, 3, 4; aspirin with codeine #2, 3, 4; Vicodin)

Codeine (Empirin): 30 mg, 60 mg round, white tablet
Tylenol: 8 mg, 15 mg, 30 mg, 60 mg round, white tablet
Vicodin: 5 mg, 500 mg capsule-shaped, white tablet

PURPOSE Moderate pain relief.

INDICATIONS For moderate, short-term pain relief.

DOSAGE The dosage of codeine is often coded by number. For example, Empirin with codeine #1 (or Empirin #1) contains one-eighth grain or 8 mg of codeine phosphate per tablet; #2 contains one-fourth grain or 16 mg; #3 contains one-half grain or 32 mg; and #4 contains 1 grain or 65 mg of codeine. A common dosage is a #3 tablet (32 mg codeine) every four hours as needed for pain.

SIDE EFFECTS The side effects are proportional to the dosage. The more you take, the more side effects you are likely to have. Allergic reactions are quite rare.

Codeine is a mild narcotic. Thus, it can lead to addiction, with tolerance and drug dependence. Frequently in older persons with arthritis it leads to constipation and sometimes a set of complications including fecal impaction and diverticulitis. More worrisome is the way that persons using codeine seem to lose their will to cope. The person taking codeine for many years sometimes seems sluggish and generally depressed. We don't really know whether the codeine is responsible, but we do think that codeine often makes it more difficult for the person with arthritis to cope with the very real problems that abound.

PERCODAN (Percobarb, Percodan-Demi, Percogesic)

Percodan: Yellow tablet
Percodan-Demi: Pink tablet

PURPOSE For pain relief.

INDICATIONS For short-term relief of moderate to severe pain.

DOSAGE One tablet every six hours as needed.

SIDE EFFECTS

Percodan is a curious combination drug. The basic narcotic is oxycodone, to which is added aspirin and other minor pain relievers. Combination drugs have a number of theoretical disadvantages, but Percodan is a strong and effective pain reliever. It does require a special prescription because it is a strong narcotic and the hazards of serious addiction are present. The manufacturers state that the habit-forming potential is somewhat less than with morphine and somewhat greater than with codeine. The drug is usually well tolerated.

SPECIAL HINTS

Percodan is a good drug for people with cancer, but it can be dangerous in the treatment of arthritis. It is not an anti-inflammatory agent and does not work directly on any of the disease processes. It is habit-forming and it does break the pain reflex. It is a mental depressant and can result in serious addiction.

DEMEROL (meperidine)

Demerol-Hydrochloride: 50 mg, 100 mg round, white, scored tablet
Demerol APAP: 50 mg tablet, pink with dark pink splotches

PURPOSE

For relief of severe pain such as in cancer, heart attacks, kidney stones.

INDICATIONS

For temporary relief of severe pain, as with a bad fracture that has been immobilized.

DOSAGE

Various preparations are available that contain 25 mg, 50 mg, or 100 mg of Demerol. One tablet every four hours for pain is a typical dose. Dose is increased for more severe pain and decreased for milder pain.

SIDE EFFECTS

Demerol is a major narcotic approximately equivalent to morphine in pain relief capacity and in addiction potential. Tolerance develops and increasing doses may be required. Drug dependence and severe withdrawal symptoms may be seen if the drug is stopped. Psychological dependence also occurs. The underlying disease may be covered up and serious symptoms may be masked. Nausea, vomiting, constipation, and a variety of other side effects may occur.

SPECIAL HINTS

This is not a drug for the treatment of arthritis. Stay away from it.

Tranquilizers

Valium, Librium, and other tranquilizers are among the most prescribed drugs in North America. They do not help arthritis. These drugs depress the patient and should be avoided by persons with arthritis whenever possible.

Muscle Relaxants

Soma, Flexeril, and a number of other agents are prescribed frequently as "muscle relaxants." In general these act like tranquilizers. They treat only symptoms and are usually not helpful in arthritis. One exception: Flexeril is sometimes useful against fibromyalgia.

Antidepressants

There is a role for antidepressant treatment in arthritis when depression is a problem, and in selected cases it can be very helpful. Sometimes a low dose of an antidepressant, such as Elavil, is given at bedtime, not to fight depression but to help improve the quality of sleep and to reduce the problems of fibromyalgia.

Hyaluronic Acid Injections (Viscosupplementation)

HYALGAN (Hyaluronan); Synvisc (Hylan G-F 20)

These two substances have recently received FDA approval for treatment of pain associated with osteoarthritis of the knee in patients who have not responded to traditional therapy. The drugs are given by injection and are intended to improve the viscosity of the synovial fluid so that lubrication in the joint is better. The injections are not inexpensive but have been shown in sound scientific experiments to be about as effective as NSAIDs.

They appear to have a role in osteoarthritis of the knee, particularly if only one knee is more severely involved. These injections appear to be similar in effectiveness to injections of corticosteroids and may prove to have fewer side effects. Still, the effects of multiple injections have not yet been studied. Relief may extend for only a few days or may last for many months, although the drug itself is present in the joint only for a few days. Medicare and many insurance companies recently have agreed to cover the initial use of these compounds. These drugs do not appear to be a major advance, but some patients will receive some benefit from them.

Alternative Medicines

Glucosamine, chondroitin sulphate

Many folk remedies are used for treatment of arthritis, and some individuals appear to benefit from some of them. Hence, it is difficult to be critical of the use of unproven or relatively unproven agents unless they are hazardous or are used in such a way as to displace the use of more effective medical treatments. In this latter case, they can be a cruel delusion.

The recent boom in the use of glucosamine and/or chondroitin sulphate is best considered an alternative medicine phenomenon. These agents are widely available over the counter, from supermarkets to health food stores. They are normal constituents of the joint cartilage and are sold as dietary supplements. There do not appear to be any major side effects. They have been used most frequently in osteoarthrosis but also have been used in a number of musculoskeletal pain syndromes.

The scientific base for the effectiveness of these compounds is currently very weak. Some quite old studies in the European medical literature suggested that they might be effective in the treatment of osteoarthritis, but most recent studies have been less impressive. It has been pointed out that there is no way these drugs could get from the stomach to the joint since they have to be broken down in the intestine into smaller molecules before they can be absorbed into the body. Hence, it is not possible for them to work by the mechanism suggested for their action. High-quality clinical studies are currently under way because of the wide use of these agents, but results are not yet available.

Many patients who take these drugs alone or together do not tell their doctor that they are taking them, largely because they fear the disapproval of the doctor. If you do take these agents, please tell your doctor, so that we can begin to build a critical medical appreciation of their effectiveness or lack of it. If any medication, whether traditional or alternative in character, appears to be giving major benefits, then it usually makes sense to continue the medication as long as benefit appears to continue. We hope to have information about the true effectiveness of these agents in the relatively near future.

Names and Availability

Some drugs are known by different names in the United States, Canada, New Zealand, Australia, and other countries. In addition, because of drugs' differing status in terms of government approval, some drugs available in one country are not available in another. For information about any drug whose name does not appear in this chapter, speak to your doctor or pharmacist.

CHAPTER 17

What About Surgery?

Surgery can relieve pain, restore function, and return a patient to employment. Its potential to satisfactorily repair a damaged joint increases year by year. But surgery is expensive and painful, is associated with a long recovery period, keeps you away from activities during the period of convalescence, and may not be successful. The joint might be worse afterward. Surgery can even kill you or paralyze you, although this is rare. The decision to undergo surgery is one that you will make with your doctor. It's a major step and you want to make the right decision. Here are some guidelines to help you sort out the issues.

General Rules

1. Surgery for arthritis is seldom urgent. With only a few exceptions, a delay of days, weeks, or even months makes relatively little difference with surgery for arthritis. If the operation is successful, you will still have the good results to enjoy; if the operation is unsuccessful, you will have delayed the pain and expense by waiting. You have plenty of time for a second opinion, or a third. You can watch your condition to see if it will go away by itself or perhaps stabilize at an acceptable level. So take your time. Rare exceptions to this rule involve bone conditions causing nerve pressure, a bacterial infection in the bone or joint, or a rupture of the tendons.

2. Not all surgeons are equal. Generally, you will want an orthopedic or hand surgeon to perform any necessary operations on your joints. You will also want a surgeon who does a lot of joint operations and is up-to-date on the latest techniques. Surgery is a rapidly changing field, and familiarity with the most recent advances leads to better results. A surgeon who performs the operation only once or twice a year is not likely to have the same level of skill as a surgeon who does the operation weekly. As a dividend, you will usually find that the busy joint surgeon is more conservative in his or her recommendation for operation. It's not at all uncommon for a good orthopedic surgeon to indicate quite candidly that the condition for which the operation is being considered is not likely to respond to surgical treatment—and then you will be spared an unsuccessful operation.

3. Not all operations are equal. Total hip replacement and total knee replacement are very fine operations; almost all patients benefit from them. On the other hand, certain procedures, such as tendon operations on the small joints of the hand or most kinds of back surgery, are far less predictable. Before you decide to have either of the latter two kinds of operation, you will want to find out how good the recommended operation is.

4. Best results are achieved when problems are localized. Treatment with medications is often best for a widespread problem. On the other hand, if the problem is localized, say to one knee, then surgery is likely to be a good, targeted approach to the problem. If a large number of joints are involved, surgery may be impractical. For example, the lower extremity has eight major weight-bearing areas: the two forefeet, the ankles, the knees, and the hips. If any one of these areas is limiting walking, surgery may be a wise move. But if all eight areas are bad, then fixing one is not going to be of particular help. Improvement in one joint without relief to the other seven cannot be expected to improve function very much. Be realistic. Ask how much better off you would be if the area of a proposed operation were entirely well. If the answer is, "Not much," then the surgery may not be advisable.

5. Best results are achieved in treatment of large joints. Joints are complicated structures, and scarring after surgery can result in stiffness, particularly if the surface area of the joint is small. The best surgical procedures repair large joints such as the hip and the knee. Results in these areas are usually predictably good. With the smaller joints, sophisticated repair techniques sometimes don't improve function significantly and should be approached with caution. Usually problems with smaller joints are also problems that involve many joints, which again complicates the surgical approach.

Specific Operations

Joint Replacement

This is the most important orthopedic surgical procedure for arthritis. The joint is removed and replaced entirely by an artificial joint. The cartilage is replaced by long-wearing plastics similar to Teflon, the bone is replaced by stainless steel, and the artificial joint is embedded in the ends of the bones on either side by a very strong cement called methyl methacralate. This bone cement first made the new era in joint surgery possible by providing a way to anchor the artificial joint to the bones.

Hip

The hip was the first joint to be "replaced." Total hip replacement is an excellent operation in the hands of an experienced surgeon. Pain is almost totally relieved and function greatly improved. The present artificial hip is estimated to last ten to fifteen years, and newer models are expected to last longer as design problems are overcome. The failure rate is only 1 or 2%. These patients may have infections or even have to have the artificial hip removed. It is true that some patients receiving artificial hips have had to have a replacement for the replacement; it is also true that this usually has been satisfactory. Recently a new type of total hip operation has been developed that works by allowing bony ingrowth into the artificial joint and that does not require cement.

Knee

The knee is a complicated hinge joint with a requirement for sideways stability. This has made it more difficult to construct an appropriate replacement joint, since the joint must move freely in the hinge direction but most strongly resist sideways force. The ball-and-socket joint of the hip poses easier engineering problems. Techniques of knee replacement have been greatly refined over the last several years and results are now very good.

Others

Ankle replacements remain less frequently used. Shoulder replacements have become quite good. Operations to replace the small joints of the fingers are widely practiced, but the outcome has not been uniformly satisfactory. One of the problems with present operations for the small joints of the hands is that appearance may be considerably improved by the straightening of deformed fingers, but the ability to use the hand may not be greatly changed.

Synovectomy

Removal of inflamed synovium is termed a synovectomy. This popular operation results in a reduction of the swelling of synovitis. Presumably there is also less enzymatic damage to the joint because the inflamed tissue mass has been reduced. Unfortunately, joint stiffness is often experienced after the synovectomy, and the inflamed tissue frequently grows back. There has been a long-standing argument about whether synovectomy should be done early or late (or never) in rheumatoid arthritis, with some doctors holding each extreme position. In other words, the effects of synovectomy are not so dramatic that people can't argue about them. There should be a special reason for this operation, such as worsening of a single joint when all other joints are in control, or the hope of avoiding the use of a hazardous drug.

Resections

Some older operations sound a bit strange, and this is the case with resection procedures. Here, bones are just cut away and removed. This sounds like it wouldn't be very helpful, but it often can be. Resection of the metatarsal heads in the forefoot, for example, can relieve pain and restore the ability to walk. Similar operations may be done in the distal ulna, the bone on the outside of the wrist. Or bunions and other protuberances can be removed. While this type of surgery is not elegant in concept, it can be very useful.

Fusion

An operation to unite two bones is termed a fusion. Such operations are useful to stabilize joints; the fusion provides a platform for movement and prevents pain in the fused area. The wrist and ankle are the joints where this procedure is most frequently used; fusion of the back or part of the neck is also performed on occasion. A successful fusion, limiting all motion, stops pain. But, in the area that is fused, flexibility is lost. Usually a fusion places additional strain on nearby joints that are called on to take over the flexibility functions. Fusion doesn't always work, and nonunion can occur. These operations are very helpful, however, every now and then.

Back Surgery

A full discussion about indications for back surgery is beyond the scope of this chapter. Most patients know from talking with friends that unsuccessful back surgery is common. In most cases the doctor was not very enthusiastic about performing this surgery, but the continuing problems of the patient eventually led doctor and patient to agree on this measure. And it didn't work.

By and large, back surgery is not advisable unless there is evidence of pressure on nerve roots. This may happen with a herniated disk, or with narrowing of the spinal canal, or with back fractures.

A myelogram can demonstrate pressure on the nerves in the spinal cord. Operations in patients with negative myelograms are the least likely to succeed. However, the myelogram itself requires placement of a needle into the spinal canal and the injection of a not-innocuous dye into the space around the spinal cord. It is uncomfortable, and there are some side effects. Hence, even considering a myelogram should be reserved for the most serious back problems.

A CT scan or magnetic resonance (MR) imaging test can provide much of the same information. The CT scan involves some radiation and is expensive, but generally safe. It doesn't hurt. Magnetic resonance (MR) imaging tests don't involve radiation. They are expensive, but they can be very helpful. The view of the back structures is extraordinarily clear.

The back is composed of an extraordinarily complex set of muscles, ligaments, and tendons. The injury may be anywhere and frequently is not in the spine itself. Hence, surgery on the spine may not be countering what is wrong. Read the sections on the back in Chapter 9, in Low Back Pain **(S12),** and in Neck Pain **(S13).** Seek multiple opinions before having a back operation. You want to avoid back surgery if you can, and it's mainly up to you.

Neurological Operations

There can be pressure on nerves in the spine or out in the limbs. An example is the carpal tunnel syndrome, where there is pressure on the nerve passing over the front of the wrist resulting in pain and tingling in the fingers. This pressure can be effectively eliminated by surgery, and surgery should be undertaken if rest and/or injection do not eliminate the syndrome within a few weeks. Other problems, such as a Morton's neuroma, can also cause peripheral pain. Here, an injury has caused the nerve fibers to grow into a little ball and to transmit pain signals all the time. If this bundle of nerves is removed, the pain is eliminated and a good result obtained. So while we can't really operate to repair nerves, we can either remove the structures that are pressing on them or remove the area that is sending the abnormal signals.

Cosmetic Surgery

We intend the term "cosmetic" here in a mildly disparaging way. Usually, surgery for a joint should be done only to relieve pain or to improve function. The appearance of the joint is much less important. Some operations serve mainly to improve appearance. Many patients are later disappointed by such operations. The appearance is less than perfect anyway, and the patient somehow had been expecting that the part would work better if it looked better, despite advice to the contrary.

CHAPTER 18

Understanding Those Tests

There are four general rules to remember about tests. First, no test is perfect. Normal people sometimes have abnormal tests, and people with arthritis often test normally. Usually these are not laboratory errors but reflect the imperfection of the test. Doctors describe tests by their *sensitivity* (ability to detect all cases) and *specificity* (ability to avoid false positives for patients who are actually normal). No test has perfect sensitivity or perfect specificity.

Second, tests do not establish the diagnosis or treatment. Rather, they confirm the impression of the physician. Any doctor who relies entirely on tests to make decisions is a bad doctor. Your doctor should have a pretty good idea of what is going on with your joints before any tests are performed; the tests will help reduce any remaining uncertainty.

Third, explanations will differ as different doctors try to make difficult concepts understandable. Don't worry if you get two quite different explanations for the same test result. Some explanations may seem absurd to the literal wordsmith, such as, "There is a little bit of arthritis in your blood"—an obvious contradiction in terms since arthritis, by definition, involves a problem with the joints, not the blood. The doctor in this instance is just trying to explain that a blood test frequently associated with arthritis is positive.

Fourth, in general, too many tests are performed. Don't demand tests or feel slighted if no tests are ordered. Often, the more experienced physician will use fewer tests. Tests for diagnosis usually don't need to be repeated after the diagnosis has been made. Tests designed to check for drug side effects or to measure improvement may need to be repeated at intervals.

In the discussion that follows, we have usually indicated (in italics) how often a test is required and how frequently, if at all, it should be repeated. These guidelines should give you a frame of reference for understanding the tests requested for your case.

The discussions are short, nontechnical, and grouped by the type of test. We have listed only the most common. The list will still seem complicated, but any individual should have only a few tests. Read about those that pertain to you.

Blood Tests

Hematocrit (PCV, Packed Cell Volume)

This test and the closely related hemoglobin test measure the number of red blood cells. The number of red blood cells will be decreased (anemia) with chronic inflammation, as in rheumatoid arthritis, and the degree of reduction corresponds to the severity of the disease. The number can also be reduced if you are losing blood through your bowel as a result of medications, or if a powerful drug has decreased the production of red cells by the bone marrow. *(Commonly employed test; often repeated frequently.)*

White Blood Count (WBC)

The white blood cells help fight infection. With infection the number is often increased, and with some drug reactions the number can be decreased. *A differential white count* will sometimes be used to determine the particular kind of white cells being increased or decreased. *(Commonly employed test; often repeated to test for drug side effects or for the possibility of infection.)*

Platelet Count

The platelets help the blood to clot. If the platelet count is too low there is a possibility of a bleeding problem. This may occur in lupus and in a few of the other diseases discussed in this book, and several of the drugs used to treat arthritis can, rarely, cause the platelet count to be very low. *(Infrequently required test; repetition frequent if the patient is taking a suspect drug.)*

Sedimentation Rate (ESR, Sed Rate)

This can be a valuable test. It tends to measure the amount of inflammation present; a high sed rate means a lot of inflammation. It can help the doctor distinguish between an inflammatory condition and a noninflammatory one. It can help determine whether the inflammation is increasing or decreasing. The test is an old and very simple one. Blood is allowed to settle in a test tube, and the distance that it settles in one hour is the sedimentation rate. If there is no inflammation, the sedimentation rate is usually less than 20 mm per hour. The C-reactive protein (CRP) test is very similar and is preferred by some doctors. (*Commonly used test; often repeated fairly frequently.*)

Blood Serum Chemistry Tests

Creatinine

This test measures how well the kidneys excrete waste products. A normal creatinine is less than 1.5 mg percent; the creatinine may rise to 10 or even 20 if kidney involvement is extremely severe. This test is generally not needed except in diseases such as lupus or polyarteritis, which may cause kidney disease. *(Infrequently required; repeated observations are necessary if there is kidney disease.)*

Liver Function Tests

Medications used for arthritis can sometimes damage the liver, and these tests are used to detect damage before it becomes severe. The tests include bilirubin (jaundice), serum albumin, and serum alkaline phosphatase. The most important, however, measure the liver enzymes SGOT (also called AST or ASAT) and SGPT (also called ALT and ALAT). These enzymes leak out of damaged liver cells and can be measured in the blood. Usually values should be below 40. With methotrexate or leflunomide therapy, they are usually measured every four to eight weeks, at least for the first one or two years, and then, if normal, perhaps less often. If they are abnormal more than half the time it can be a signal to reduce the dose or even to consider a liver biopsy to check for serious damage. The anti-inflammatory drugs (NSAIDs), especially aspirin and Voltaren, can also cause (usually minor) effects on these tests but do not require regular monitoring in most people. *(Required only with methotrexate, leflunomide, or perhaps Imuran treatment, although occasionally testing is part of a general checkup. For monitoring, regular testing is needed.)*

Blood Serum Immunology Tests

Latex (Rheumatoid Factor, RF)

Many patients with rheumatoid arthritis have a large amount of *rheumatoid factor* circulating in their blood. This factor is also found in patients with no disease at all and in patients with other diseases, although less frequently than in rheumatoid arthritis. A latex test isn't worth much unless it has a *titer* associated with it. The titer tells how much of the rheumatoid factor is present. Patients with rheumatoid arthritis usually have a titer of 1:160 or greater. Some other diseases also can cause high titers. The rheumatoid factor titer is sometimes used to document improvement, but it actually isn't very useful for this. Recently many laboratories have changed this test and now report results in "International Units." A result of over 40 units is considered abnormal, and results can go up to 2,000 units or more. *(Required fairly frequently for diagnosis; should be repeated infrequently.)*

Antinuclear Antibody Tests (ANA, FANA)

Antinuclear antibodies can be found in normal individuals, particularly with increasing age. However, they are almost always present in patients with lupus and are often found in patients with rheumatoid arthritis or other connective-tissue diseases. If the ANA is negative, a diagnosis of lupus is unlikely. Warning: These tests are often overinterpreted and cause unnecessary concern. A positive test doesn't necessarily mean disease. A positive test can be caused by drugs or just by the aging process. A high titer increases the chance of lupus or a related disease, and doctors get some additional information from the *pattern of fluorescence. (ANA tests are required infrequently and do not require frequent repeat testing because values change very slowly.)*

DNA (Anti-DNA, DNA Binding Test)

Several tests measure antibody to DNA, an important body protein. Antibody to DNA is found almost exclusively in the disease lupus. In lupus, if the amount of DNA antibody rises, the situation is potentially more severe. *(Required in very few patients, essentially only those with lupus, but some such patients may require testing as often as monthly.)*

ENA (Extractable Nuclear Antibody)

This test measures an antibody to an antigen that is found in connective-tissue diseases and is characteristic of an unusual syndrome called MCTD or mixed connective-tissue disease, which combines features of myositis, lupus, and scleroderma. When this syndrome is present, a very high titer to the ENA is often found, perhaps as high as 1:100,000 or 1:1,000,000. The anti-RNP on anti-Sm tests can help determine what kind of ENA is present. *(Infrequently required; since it changes only very slowly, repeat tests are seldom required.)*

Complement (C-3, C-4, CH50)

The complement proteins tend to be reduced when lupus is active. The normal and abnormal values vary depending on the laboratory and the particular technique used. *(Required in few patients, essentially only those patients with lupus, but may then be repeated periodically.)*

Tissue-typing Tests

B27 (HLA-B27)

Tissue-typing tests originally were developed to improve the results in organ transplantation, such as of the kidneys or heart. As a by-product, the fascinating relationship between the B27 tissue type and attachment arthritis was discovered. This arthritis runs in families and is found in some of those family members who have the B27 gene. The gene is transmitted by either the father or mother, and approximately one-half of the children will have the gene. In some instances this test can help in the diagnosis of arthritis. The tissue type is similar to the familiar blood type, but it is done by typing the white cells rather than the red cells. *(Infrequently required, and only when there is suspicion of an attachment arthritis; test needs not be repeated since tissue type does not change.)*

Urine Tests

Urinalysis

This is actually a number of tests. In the area of the rheumatic diseases doctors often look for red blood cells, protein, or casts in the urine. These findings suggest nephritis (kidney inflammation) and are sometimes encountered in lupus or arteritis. In addition, drugs such as gold and penicillamine can cause protein loss through the urine. Normal urine has very few red blood cells, no urine protein, and no casts. *(Frequently employed; may be repeated in diseases where kidney involvement is possible or with a drug, such as gold salts or penicillamine, that might cause kidney damage.)*

24-Hour Urine Tests (24-Hour Protein; 24-Hour Creatinine Clearance)

These tests determine how much of a particular compound is excreted in 24 hours. All urine excreted in a full day is collected. This can give a more accurate estimate of the amount of protein leakage, and the *creatinine clearance* can give an accurate measure of kidney function. Creatinine is a chemical compound found in blood, urine, and muscle. The creatinine clearance is calculated from the blood creatinine value and the 24-hour urine creatinine. This is a cumbersome way to measure kidney function, but it is preferred by some doctors to the serum creatinine value alone. *(The 24-hour protein test will be used only when a routine urinalysis shows that there is some protein leakage. The 24-hour creatinine clearance may be obtained as a "baseline" in a disease where kidney disease is possible and may be repeated at intervals.)*

Biopsies

Skin Biopsy

A small piece of skin may be removed and examined under the microscope to confirm a diagnosis of scleroderma or of some forms of arteritis. It may be used to confirm a diagnosis of lupus, psoriasis, or other skin conditions. The procedure is virtually painless and leaves a small scar. It is done under local anesthesia, very quickly, and does not require hospitalization. *(Usually does not need to be repeated.)*

Kidney Biopsy (Renal Biopsy)

This procedure is more hazardous than the skin biopsy. Through a needle inserted in the back, a small core of kidney tissue is removed and examined under the microscope. Complications, particularly bleeding, can occur; blood transfusions are required after 1 to 3% of kidney biopsies. Death has resulted, but it is exceedingly rare. Very rarely, the bleeding may require removal of the kidney. There is controversy about how frequently these tests should be performed. I use them rarely; some other doctors use them more frequently. *(Rarely needs to be repeated.)*

Muscle Biopsy

Biopsy of the muscle is a safe and easy procedure resulting in a small scar; it is a little more difficult than a skin biopsy. Sometimes skin and muscle biopsies are done together. The muscle biopsy finds its greatest value in the diagnosis of polymyositis or dermatomyositis, or in the documentation of inflammation in the arteries (arteritis). *(Rarely needs to be repeated.)*

Temporal Artery Biopsy

In this biopsy a piece of the artery that runs across the temple is removed. One or both temporal arteries may be biopsied. This biopsy is simple and has few complications. It can be useful in the diagnosis of giant-cell (temporal) arteritis and is sometimes performed in polymyalgia rheumatica (PMR). It sounds like a major procedure to cut out a piece of an artery, but the scalp is so well supplied with blood vessels that you really don't need this one. Some patients who have headaches related to temporal artery inflammation actually get relief from their headaches after the biopsy. *(Used only when there is a suspicion of giant-cell arteritis, temporal arteritis, or PMR, and not always needed even then. Rarely needs to be repeated.)*

Liver Biopsy

This procedure is sometimes recommended for patients who have been taking methotrexate for a long time and who have abnormal liver blood tests. Usually it will not be needed. It is discussed in the section on methotrexate treatment (pages 150–151). *(Rarely needs to be repeated.)*

Joint Fluid Tests

A needle can be placed into a joint in order to remove joint fluid for laboratory analysis. The procedure is generally easy, particularly in the knee, does not require hospitalization, and has only rare complications (infection is the most common). Complications are slightly higher if a substance is injected into the joint.

This test seems like such a direct way to get information about arthritis that it is disappointing that it isn't of more use. It is required if the doctor suspects infection in the joint space, since the particular bacteria can be cultured and identified. It is highly useful if crystal arthritis is suspected and a firm diagnosis has not been made, because identification of the crystals absolutely proves that a crystal arthritis is present. (Occasionally a crystal arthritis is present although the crystals are not seen.) Examination of the joint fluid can assist in determining whether the arthritis is extremely inflammatory or not. However, the tests performed on the fluid, including cell counts, joint fluid sugar level, mucin clot tests, and protein measurement, do not absolutely distinguish one kind of arthritis from another except with positive identification of crystals or bacteria.

X-rays

In general, be cautious about X-rays; you are probably aware of the hazards of radiation exposure. There is a popular impression that X-rays give doctors much more information than they actually do. Only the bony structures are well seen on X-rays; problems that affect "soft" tissues of the body don't really show up. The doctor can often tell by examination exactly what would be revealed by an X-ray, so the X-ray doesn't contribute anything. Further, changes to bone sometimes take several years to develop; if the arthritis hasn't persisted for a long time, it's possible that the X-ray examination will be normal. The critical question in any test that involves expense or hazard is whether it will add any information to that which is already known. X-rays are requested by patients too often, and many patients seem disappointed if the doctor does not recommend X-rays.

Hand X-rays

These X-rays may be obtained every couple of years in rheumatoid and some other forms of arthritis to determine the rate of bony destruction, if any. Severe rheumatoid arthritis causes small holes near the ends of the bones, and the increase in extent of these erosions is a measure of disease progression. Psoriatic arthritis shows a strange "whittled" appearance in some cases, and osteoarthritis shows narrowing of the joint spaces and development of bone spurs.

Sacroiliac X-rays

X-rays of the sacroiliac joints are important in ankylosing spondylitis, which is defined as including damage to the sacroiliac joints. Without this X-ray, the diagnosis cannot be made. The X-ray examination of the sacroiliac joints is more important than the B27 test or other findings that suggest ankylosing spondylitis. After a year or so of ankylosing spondylitis, the margins of the sacroiliac joints begin to blur, and the bone becomes a bit more dense near the joint. Later, the joint space narrows. In advanced disease the joint entirely disappears, with bone replacing what used to be the sacroiliac joint. These joints are seldom involved in ordinary low back syndromes or in other kinds of arthritis, so these X-rays are usually required only in patients with suspected attachment arthritis. I prefer to get a single X-ray film of the pelvis to inspect the sacroiliac joints because I am able to see a little bit of the hip joints and the lower spine as well. Some doctors prefer to get special angled pictures of the sacroiliac joints themselves.

Cervical Spine (C-Spine) X-rays

Neck views are frequently requested for osteoarthritis, particularly if pain from the neck extends into the arms or there is weakness in the hands. The doctor is looking for narrowing of the holes through which the nerves pass and for narrowing of the disks. Unfortunately, the X-rays can be pretty confusing. Many patients with narrowed holes for the nerves have no problem whatsoever; others with problems have relatively normal X-rays. Rheumatoid arthritis can affect the upper one or two vertebrae in the spine, just at the base of the skull, and juvenile arthritis also can affect the neck.

Lumbar Spine (L-Spine) X-rays

Low back syndromes, unless they have been recurrent or are associated with nerve symptoms, don't routinely require X-rays. If a disk problem is suspected, some information may be obtained by a plain X-ray, although, like the cervical spine X-ray, the results can be confusing. Many patients have symptoms without much abnormality, and other patients have a lot of abnormality without any symptoms. The myelogram, a more extensive X-ray in which dye is injected into the spinal canal, is more accurate in identifying nerve pressure. A CT scan or MR imaging test can also visualize these areas well. In attachment arthritis, the lumbar spine can be involved, and X-rays can depict the degree of involvement. This X-ray is overused and is often done only because patients (or lawyers) seem to expect it.

Areas of Pain and Discomfort

Almost any part of the body can be X-rayed. Calcium deposits may be located in the shoulder X-ray, arthritis in the feet may be investigated, and problems in the knees, hips, or other joints can be examined. It doesn't usually make much sense to X-ray areas that aren't painful since they are usually normal. And if the pain hasn't been present for very long, a normal X-ray is likely. Finally, treatment for most local conditions, such as tennis elbow, isn't likely to be improved by an X-ray. A good practice is to let your doctor suggest the X-ray—don't bring up the subject yourself.

CHAPTER 19

Duck That Quack

Over one-half of people with significant arthritis are victimized by one or another confidence game at some point. Usually the person who receives quack treatments has seen a physician first, so to some extent the existence of quackery reflects a failure of traditional medicine to set proper expectations and to deliver hope. When I ask a patient why he or she went to some improbable healer, the answer is usually, "The doctors didn't seem to be able to do anything." People don't like to have a chronic disease, don't like to be told that they have to do some of the work toward a cure, and don't like to learn that the answer is not simple. The trademark of the phony treatment is the promise of a simple, easy, and exclusive cure. Unfortunately, it is *never* that easy.

What Do You Have to Lose?

What's the harm? If a quack treatment isn't dangerous, why not give it a try? (And it usually isn't dangerous, with a few notable exceptions described below. For obvious reasons, a quack treatment that directly harms people won't last long.) What do you have to lose from the quack? More than you think. You have to consider the issues carefully to understand all that has been lost. Among the losses are: money, courage, will, patience, confidence, dignity, function, life.

Money is the most obvious loss to quackery and has been estimated at several hundred million dollars a year in the United States alone. The cost can range from a few dollars for a quack book or a copper bracelet to many thousands of dollars for fraudulent injections or heavily promoted spa treatments. Many arthritis frauds make a lot of visible money for somebody, be it an author, a practitioner, or an institution. This is *your* money.

Since others would quickly adopt any treatment that truly helped a lot of people, a gimmick being used by only one or two practitioners is highly suspect.

Courage and will are precious attributes for the patient with arthritis, and they are eroded by the disillusionment experienced when a false cure fails. Quack treatment failures can make it even more difficult for arthritis sufferers to have the patience demanded by valid treatment programs.

Confidence is closely related to courage and will. If you have confidence in your doctor, you will do better than if you don't. A pattern of rejection of any suggestion made by the doctor is often a vicious aftermath of quack treatment. Losses of courage, will, patience, and confidence have to do with loss of the spirit.

Dignity is another profound loss. You were taken in. You were the mark. Somebody manipulated you. You were taken advantage of. You were gullible, stupid, suckered, ripped off. Your pride, integrity, and autonomy are shaken. Perhaps you overcompensate by clinging to a belief in the fraud even after it fails. You rationalize. Trying to salvage your dignity, you may even tell your friends that it worked.

Displacement of sound treatment by a fraudulent treatment can result in disability or death. Even if you tell yourself that the quack treatment will be in addition to sound treatment, this is unlikely to hold true. Confidence in the sound treatment is apt to be undermined by the self-promotion of the quack treatment. For example, one widely distributed quack book tells patients not to take gold treatments; it's hard to know how much damage has been done by this advice, but it must be considerable. A patient of mine stopped good treatment for her systemic lupus after quack advice, and the chain of events that followed led to the loss of function of both her kidneys and one eye.

Direct side effects of quack treatments can lead to death. Prednisone and phenylbutazone given by quack promoters have caused fatalities and major complications. Mexican-border clinics have been the source of many of these prescriptions. A particular Chinese herb causes liver damage in some patients.

The terms *quack* and *fraud* are used in this chapter to refer to treatments that lack a rationale acceptable to scientific consensus and that are not supported by acceptable evidence for effectiveness. In other words, there is no reason to think they should work and no evidence that they do. I do not mean to imply by use of these strong words that all quack practitioners have self-serving, malicious intentions; some sincerely believe in their treatments. I also do not intend to ascribe omniscience to the present scientific consensus, which is likely to be in error in a variety of ways we do not yet suspect.

However, I follow about 2,000 patients with various forms of arthritis. About 20%, to my knowledge, have used a quack treatment at some point. A few have reported some degree of temporary improvement; the rest have bitterly described failure. I have never seen a beneficial response from such treatment that wasn't to be expected without the treatment. I have personally observed repeated failures and adverse complications from unorthodox treatments.

The Written Word as Quackery

Supermarkets and newsstands carry publications that remain technically short of pure fantasy but distort minor therapeutic advances into dramatic curative breakthroughs. There is usually some tenuous basis for the story, and sometimes the authorities cited are actually experts of considerable stature. The "arthritis cure" headline is repeated every four to six months, always with a different cure.

Usually the headlines are more misleading than the content of the article, but all tricks are used. The sensational part is on the front page; only after purchasing the paper do you turn to the far less sensational information on the inside. Old information is treated as new, slight changes are described as dramatic, and quotations are taken out of context. The articles are sensational, simplistic, quick, and easy. They tell you what you want to believe. Every such issue wastes a lot of doctor time and patient concern by necessitating discussion and explanation of the nonissues raised.

Quack books may employ a similar sales tactic. The title is likely to contain the words *safe, easy,* or *cure.* There is generally a single, rather thin gimmick purported to be the author's discovery after years of "research"; the rest of the book is padding around the gimmick. There may be an M.D. or D.O. as author, or there may be a preface by an M.D. or a D.O. The treatment is "proved effective" on the basis of letters received, and portions of letters are sometimes included in the text. If there is any reference to the scientific medical literature, most references are to the 1920–1970 period.

I have reviewed every such book that I could find. The gimmicks employed include cod-liver oil, eating foods in the right order, frequent enemas, vinegar and honey diets, vitamin C, vitamin D, vitamin E, vitamin A, glucosamine, chondroitin sulphate, and others. If the subject were not so serious, the explanations developed would be amusing. One suggests, for example, that glucosamine will "oil" the joints, although it is impossible for glucosamine to be absorbed into the body without first being broken apart by the digestive system. Such theories are an insult to the intelligence of the reader. Avoid all books with the simplistic formula described above. Look for favorable mention by the Arthritis Foundation or the Arthritis Society, by the National Institutes of Health or other governmental bodies, or by scientists from major universities.

Some Well-publicized "Cures"

Flu shots Yep, three flu shots cure arthritis, and you can get them in California for a fee. These clever doctors are entirely legal and even have you sign a paper saying that you were not told the shots would cure your arthritis.

Bee stings Bee-venom desensitization cures arthritis, according to several doctors; for a fee, they will give you a series of injections. This is a carry-over from a treatment popular many years ago—before it was discarded as worthless.

Border-clinic pills Several "clinics" exist in Mexican border towns that attract considerable United States money. This is probably the most malignant arthritis fraud being perpetrated at the present time. Pills supplied by these clinics are dangerous and have killed people. The dispensers lie about the content of the pills. The pills contain a corticosteroid and sometimes other dangerous medications like phenylbutazone, but the dispensers deny this even when directly questioned. I have had pills from these clinics analyzed on more than 12 occasions, and each time the analysis found a cortisone-like drug. These pills give days of relief and years of consequences.

Elsewhere in Mexico there are fine physicians of high principle who are genuinely expert in the management of patients with rheumatic diseases. The indictment above is not meant to criticize all medical care in Mexico but, rather, specific fraudulent clinics operating along the United States–Mexico border.

Uranium mines Fortunately, tests with Geiger counters have shown that these potentially dangerous mines don't even have any radiation. Medically, while the use of focused lymphoid radiation in rheumatoid arthritis is still being debated, all agree that total body irradiation is harmful and dangerous.

Copper bracelets Just kind of silly.

Antifungus treatment Arthritis is seen as an allergic reaction to a fungus, to be cured by antifungal drugs. They don't work.

Elimination diets Arthritis is seen as a result of food allergy. Following a period of fasting, groups of foods are reintroduced into the diet. There are some well-meaning people who believe in this, but all scientific studies have been negative. Unfortunately this "clinical ecology" approach, particularly in rheumatoid arthritis, often results in a serious delay in obtaining effective treatment.

Acupuncture The acupuncture fad arrived at a time when political barriers against exchange with China were decreasing. In our haste to welcome Chinese wisdom back into the world community, we overlooked some rather basic observations. Acupuncture has a long and noble history in China and has been developed for uses that are alien to our Western appreciation. For example, acupuncture is used to some extent as anesthesia for surgical operations.

However, acupuncture is not used for the treatment of rheumatoid arthritis in China and is felt by Chinese acupuncturists to be ineffective for this purpose. It is used in China for treatment of certain local conditions. In our haste to accept acupuncture we invented uses that had long since been discarded by the societies we were trying to court. Several good scientific studies were done in the United States to determine the usefulness of acupuncture for rheumatoid arthritis and osteoarthritis, particularly of the knees. The studies showed no effect on arthritis, although one study showed a slight decrease in pain, rather less than with aspirin.

Acupressure An ingenious, timely, novel, and worthless extrapolation of acupuncture.

Glucosamine and/or chondroitin sulphate These "food supplements" are widely promoted and widely available, and are described in Chapter 16. While they have not been proved worthless yet, they cannot work by the mechanism postulated since they cannot get into the joint; they are broken down by the digestive system first. They are promoted simplistically as cure-alls and may sometimes displace adherence to good medical recommendations.

And then there is Madison Avenue

- *"More of the pain reliever doctors recommend most."* Translation: Simple aspirin, overpriced.

- *"Extra-strength formula." "Arthritis formula."* Translation: Larger pills.
- *"As much pain relief as you can get without a doctor's prescription."* Translation: Overpriced aspirin, acetaminophen, naproxen, or ibuprofen.
- *"The pain reliever hospitals use most."* Translation: The drug company supplies it to the hospitals at cost so that it can make the claim.

Since these claims are technically factual, the advertising is technically legal. Perhaps we need a sales boycott by consumers of medicines that are marketed in a misleading way. It is often hard even to read the ingredients of many over-the-counter pain medicines. There is no medical reason of which I am aware why you should buy any of the most heavily advertised over-the-counter products for arthritis. Less expensive products with the same ingredients often will save you money—and you will be taking a stand for honesty in product promotion.

CHAPTER 20

Saving Money Safely

Health is more important than money, but you need money too. You don't want to let the notion that "nothing is too much for my health" lead you into blindly purchasing medical goods or services you could equally well purchase for substantially less. Nor do you want "insurance will cover it" to keep you from being as careful with your medical purchases as you are with your other purchases. We pay the insurance premiums, and we all have the obligation to keep them as low for ourselves as we can. Your taxes, which pay a big chunk of medical expenses, are related to the medical bills you and others run up. Regardless of who pays the bill now, *you* pay it over the long term.

This chapter is about saving money without sacrificing health—hence, the title. The suggestions offered in this chapter can save you 50% or more on the costs of your arthritis treatment. Only a few of these suggestions may apply to you or your family, but use the ones that apply, after checking with your doctor.

Saving Money on Medications

Take as few medications as possible. "Polypharmacy" is usually an indication of less-than-optimal medical care. Ask the doctor if all the medications are necessary. Problems with multiple medications include: increased likelihood of side effects from at least one; potential ill effects from the chemical interactions between the different drugs; and the small amount of benefit that is likely to accrue—if three drugs don't fix you up, four are unlikely to do the trick. The perceptive patient or physician usually seeks to substitute one medication for another if a program is not going well, rather than adding a new drug.

Take medication as directed. "Saving pills" is false economy and may impair your health and ultimately be more costly. Some pills can be taken as you feel you need them; many must be taken very regularly. Check with your doctor. If you don't follow instructions your doctor may not be able to evaluate correctly the cause of your problem and the effectiveness of prescribed medication. Additional expensive medication may be prescribed. As a consequence, your health may be adversely affected.

Throw out old medications. Anything over three years old should go—earlier if it is past the expiration date on the package. Saving old medications is false economy.

Use generic medications whenever possible. These are medicines sold by their chemical name rather than the brand name, and they are not protected by patent. So competitive prices make them less expensive. Ask your doctor if a generic medication is possible. For example, prednisone (a generic drug) costs only one-tenth to one-twentieth as much as Medrol, Decadron, Aristocort, and other steroids bought by brand name. Yet prednisone is the best understood of all these drugs. Indocin and Naprosyn are available in generic formulations as indomethacin and naproxen; Motrin is available generically as ibuprofen. Ibuprofen and naproxen are also available in over-the-counter brand names—Advil and Nuprin for ibuprofen, Aleve for naproxen. Unfortunately, these brand-name products may be even more expensive than the corresponding prescription drugs.

Don't request "new" drugs. Usually your expectations for such drugs are unrealistically high, and these agents are always expensive. Your doctor will suggest a new drug to you if it seems to have particular promise.

Avoid unnecessary drugs. Know the purpose of each drug you take, and make sure it makes sense. For example, allopurinol and probenecid are frequently prescribed for asymptomatic hyperuricemia, a minor laboratory abnormality that isn't even a disease. Patients may spend $400 or more a year for life as a result of such unnecessary prescriptions. Other situations in which drugs might be unnecessary are long-term treatment for local conditions or treatment during asymptomatic periods. Check with your doctor as to whether the medication need be continued.

Minimize the use of painkillers. Darvon, Talwin, codeine, Percodan, Empirin #3, Tylenol #3, and so forth have a very limited role in treatment of arthritis. Avoid these when possible, and take as few as possible if you take any at all.

Minimize the use of tranquilizers and mood drugs. Amphetamines, Dexamyl, Valium, Librium, Dalmane, and a variety of other best-selling agents that lift you up, put you down, or keep you asleep have a very limited role in the management of arthritis. Avoid such drugs whenever possible, and take as few as possible.

Avoid combination drugs. You seldom need all of the elements of a combination drug, just as you don't usually need many separate drugs. In the combination drug, the proportion of the drugs is fixed and flexibility is lost. You pay for the unneeded ingredients in increased costs and side effects.

Avoid heavily advertised drugs. Excedrin, Anacin, Empirin, Ascriptin, and Arthritis Pain Formula, among others, have no advantage and some disadvantages over standard preparations. They may cost five to ten times as much. There is seldom a reason to buy these drugs for your arthritis.

Watch out for injections. By and large, injections of painkillers or cortisone into joints or ligaments should be performed sparingly. Usually, simpler things should be tried first, and injection into a painful area shouldn't be repeated more than a few times. It is all right to question your doctor if he or she suggests what seems to be too many injections. Sometimes they are needed, often not.

Saving Money on Laboratory Tests

Don't ask for trouble by requesting tests, expecting them, or being disappointed if none are ordered. The best doctors are very selective in ordering tests. Patient requests are a major reason for performance of some very doubtful procedures. You can keep the pressure off.

Keep records of previous tests, and bring the results to your doctor. Avoid the expensive repetition of laboratory work that has already been performed. A major reason for ordering laboratory tests is simply that records have been lost or are unavailable.

Some laboratory tests should be repeated periodically throughout an illness; some should not. Check Chapter 18 to get some feeling for how often a particular test should be ordered. Don't repeat tests that have value only the first time.

Laboratory test schedules can often be simplified. For example, if you are having tests of blood and urine to detect toxicity from gold injections, there are several acceptable means for the doctor to check for toxicity. The simplest ones cost about $600 to $800 for a 20-week initial course of gold, just for the laboratory testing. This is costly enough, but the more complicated schedules offer no additional safety and cost $1,000 or more. Ask your doctor to check on his or her schedule.

Can you do it yourself? Some laboratory tests, such as urinalysis, can be performed at home without special training or much expense. Patients with diabetes do it all the time by testing the urine with a piece of test paper that turns color to indicate the contents of the urine. If your urine is being checked regularly to monitor for drug side effects, you may want to check it yourself at home and keep a chart to bring to the doctor.

Can you have it done closer to home? Transportation and your time are hidden costs involved in laboratory testing. You may be able to save significantly in both areas if you can find a good laboratory with a more convenient location. Laboratories will release results to you if so instructed by your physician, or the results can be mailed directly to the doctor.

Saving Money on X-rays and Imaging Tests

Again, don't ask for trouble. Patient requests are a major reason for performance of X-rays that have limited medical value. X-rays involve radiation, although the amount is small; they also cost money, and this amount often is not small. Let the doctor suggest X-rays, CT scans, or MR imaging if necessary. CT and MR scans are not often needed for arthritis.

One X-ray or several? For X-rays of the hands, feet, and the sacroiliac joints, often one picture is as useful as several different views. The cost differential is considerable. Check with the doctor to see if several views are required, and if not, request the simpler procedure. Less radiation and less cost are both desirable.

Be especially careful with major X-rays—the upper GI (gastrointestinal) series, the barium enema, the arteriogram, and so forth. These are expensive, uncomfortable procedures, they take a good bit of time, and they may, in rare instances, cause you some difficulty. They aren't required very often for arthritis, and you ought to be sure that you understand the need for them if they are ordered.

Repeat X-rays are not needed very often. Usually the interval should be at least one year between X-ray examinations, and five years is often the more appropriate interval. If infection is suspected the doctor may need X-rays more frequently, but make sure you understand the need for frequent repeat X-rays.

Get your previous X-rays. It takes a little bit of work to pry your old X-rays out of the file room where they are stored so you can take them to a new health facility. But it is well worth the hassle. You don't want X-rays repeated just because the old ones aren't readily available.

Question the *skeletal survey.* It is very easy for the doctor to order a skeletal survey, which is an X-ray of essentially all of the bones of the body. In arthritis, only certain areas of the body will be of real interest on the X-ray. The extra expense and radiation from the additional X-ray films can be safely avoided.

The imaging tests, CT and MR, are expensive and are greatly over-performed in the United States (for example, they are used only one-tenth as often in Canada). They usually are not necessary in arthritis, and you should get a good, convincing explanation before you have one. The most frequent exceptions are presurgical, for sports injuries, and to check for narrowing of the spinal canal.

Saving Money on Doctor Visits

Get a doctor—one doctor, in whom you have confidence. If you and your doctor don't get along, change doctors, but change early rather than often. Doctor shopping and doctor switching waste time, money, and health.

Don't go to the doctor too soon. Refer to the chart on page 5 and those in Part III for instructions about the appropriate interval between initial concern and a visit to the doctor.

Don't go too often. Work out the needed frequency of visits with your physician. Consider this: If you go to the doctor every three weeks, it costs twice as much as it does to go every six weeks. Even less expensive may be an arrangement where you call for an appointment if a problem needs attention. Decisions about how often to see a patient are often made casually without much thought about what the exact interval should be. There is often lots of room for discussion, so ask your doctor. In some locations a nurse practitioner can help with routine problems at less cost.

Duck the quack. Chapter 19 suggests ways to avoid funneling your money into the pockets of those waiting to exploit you.

Ask for a second opinion. If you have doubts about a big decision your doctor recommends, check it out. It costs a little extra to be certain, but you may be able to avoid the procedure altogether. This is often important for surgical decisions and sometimes for large medical decisions, such as institution of treatment with gold salts, immunosuppressants, or penicillamine. If a liver biopsy is suggested before you start methotrexate treatment, get a second opinion. You can use this book as a second opinion, and then decide if you need a third opinion. This saves money.

Question referrals you don't understand. If your doctor is referring you too frequently, you may be better off with a specialist who knows how to manage your problems. If too many consultations and referrals are needed, your care can become expensive and fragmented. A *rheumatologist* is also a specialist in internal medicine and usually can help with your general medical problems as well.

Saving Money on Hospitals

Don't go into the hospital unless it is essential. There are relatively few reasons for hospitalization of the patient with arthritis. Among the doubtful indications are hospitalization for uncomplicated low back syndromes, for biopsy procedures, because of a bad home situation, or for a series of tests. Usually another solution that is less expensive, less time-consuming, and equally good for you can be found in such circumstances. If you do enter the hospital for a "borderline" reason, the insurance company may sometimes refuse to pay some or all of the costs. If you work effectively with your doctor on your home program, you usually should do well and not require hospitalization.

Look for facilities at lower cost. Increasingly hospitals offer a range of services for patients with different kinds of problems. The intensive care unit may now cost $2,000 per day, but facilities where you do some self-care may be available at much lower cost. You might want to consider them.

Go home soon. Hospitalizations often drag along beyond "MHB"—maximal hospital benefit. Often this is because the patient exerts pressure on the physician to stay in the hospital a few extra days. This is not a healthy habit for you; as soon as you are able, go home.

Have procedures scheduled before admission. Preadmission testing is possible in many hospitals and can decrease the stay by a day or more. If you have surgery, go into the hospital for the minimum time required before the procedure is scheduled.

Avoid hospitalization during a weekend if you can. The hospital slows down over the weekend; the laboratory and other facilities are not staffed as completely. If a weekend intervenes in your hospitalization, it may result in a couple of wasted days.

Understand and question. This is really the point of all the suggestions above. The world is changing. Good doctors and good clinics will understand your financial questions. As an intelligent consumer you have the right to agree or disagree with those things that are being done for you and to you. Pose your questions thoughtfully, and work out solutions that are comfortable for both you and the doctor. Arthritis care can be very expensive. Your problem may last many months or even many years. It may involve expenses in all of the areas discussed above, and it may impact your ability to remain employed. Protection of your financial security is an essential element of good medical treatment. Personal bankruptcy is not conducive to improved health. The impact of nonmedical factors, such as personal finances, on medical outcome is increasingly recognized. The good physician will be sympathetic and helpful with your financial problems.

CHAPTER 21

Preventing Arthritis

Perhaps you don't have arthritis (yet). Or your family and friends see your arthritis and want to know what they can do to protect themselves. Just as it is important to take preventive measures against heart disease and cancer, it is important to prevent problems with the bones, joints, and muscles. As you get older, you need reserve strength in your heart muscle. You also need reserve strength in your muscles and joints. The techniques for preventing arthritis are simple but not easy. You have to work at them. There is a big bonus, however. By maintaining a lifestyle healthy for arthritis, you also protect your heart, and the measures you need to protect against arthritis will make you feel better, will give you more energy, will improve the quality of your life, and can even extend your life. So there are rewards for the hard work. The three major things you need to do are: keep fit, control your weight, and protect your joints.

Keep Fit

Exercise has many benefits. First, our bones increase in strength—use of our bones causes the calcium content to increase and the tissues that support our weight to thicken. Ligaments tighten and become thicker with use, providing better support for the joint structures. Cartilage is nourished by motion of the joint, which brings oxygen into the cartilage and takes the waste products out. For arthritis prevention you need strong bones, strong supporting ligaments, and healthy cartilage. Exercise is the way to get these.

Exercise for arthritis prevention must be a regular part of your life. It should be repeated daily. Your exercise program should be expanded only very slowly from your beginning level. Plan to maintain your healthy habits for the rest of your life. There is no hurry. Slow and steady does it.

Great strength doesn't help. Weight lifting, push-ups, pull-ups, and so forth are not of great benefit. Repetitious but less strenuous activities such as walking, biking, and swimming are superb. The muscles gain tone, the bones gain strength, and the ligaments gain both flexibility and strength. Start with walking, bicycling, or swimming. After you're in shape, jogging, tennis, handball, soccer, or basketball are all acceptable forms of activity. But don't start off with high-intensity exercises before your ligaments and bones have had a number of months of more gentle exercise progression. Minor injuries are common in the first months of a program. Sports such as football and baseball are not particularly good exercise, and they aren't often practical for lifelong programs anyway.

Start off slowly. If you do not have a major medical problem there is little point in a complete physical examination before exercising. After all, you're just going to be doing what the body was designed to do. If you have questions, mention to your doctor that you are in the process of starting a gradual exercise progression. Plan on at least 5 days a week, and at least 12 to 15 minutes of steady exercise each day. Your goal, which may take a year or more to achieve, is to have a morning resting pulse rate of less than 60 beats per minute. If you achieve this, you have good health, good cardiac reserve, and almost certainly have strengthened your musculoskeletal system to resist the aging process.

Common sense is the essential element. You can continue to increase your activity to any desired level, including marathon running, mountain climbing, or other dramatic examples of intensive physical activity. But getting the benefits of exercise does *not* require heroic exercise programs. Every bit helps; the essential element is that a program be enjoyable and regular for life. It may take some time before you feel comfortable and easy about exercise, for old habits are hard to break. The euphoria that many exercisers report may not be experienced until the second or third year of a program. But you will have more zip in the evenings after only a few weeks or months. Health is its own reward.

Control Your Weight

Being overweight has many bad effects that we tend to forget.

- The extra weight places unnecessary stress on our weight-bearing joints.
- The tendons and ligaments become separated by layers of fat, so the leverage designed into your muscles and ligaments can't be smoothly applied. This results in more effort for a given task and creates tension

on the ligament attachments from a direction for which they were not designed. Episodes of bursitis and tendinitis are likely to result.

- Fat people are less active, although they often hate to admit it.
- Certain arthritis syndromes are much more common in the overweight. Low back pain is considerably more common in people who are obese, and some low back pain problems result from herniation of fat globules through back tissues. Some doctors feel that people with high triglycerides and high cholesterol develop certain kinds of arthritis. Surgery for obesity that bypasses the intestine can cause an arthritis.
- Other fat-related diseases limit activity. These include diabetes, hernias, hemorrhoids, gallbladder problems, and even arteriosclerosis.

Weight control also requires lifetime discipline. You first need to establish your desired weight and set your long-term goals. Then, basically, you need to eat less. The number of calories you take in must correspond with the calories you burn. You need to set intermediate goals for weight loss, and you should integrate your exercise program with your weight-control program. Keep a graph of your progress toward your goals, and achieve the goals on time. When you reach that bottom line, buy yourself new clothes and continue the graph, keeping your weight within five pounds (2 kg) of where you want to be. Expect some musculoskeletal pains during the weight-reduction phase and during the first few months at your ideal weight. These result from the tightening of the ligaments to the new dimensions of your body. They will go away and you will feel better. Don't let your weight go up and down like a yo-yo. Establish your desired weight, and control it at that level.

Are you fat? Look in the mirror. Don't be overly concerned about meeting current norms for the ideal or "fashionable" weight. If you pinch the flesh around your middle and there is more than an inch (2.5 cm) between your thumb and forefinger, you are fat. And when you look in the mirror without any clothes on, it is hard to avoid the proper conclusion. Fight the tendency to rationalize ("I don't eat a thing"; "I have big bones"). You know better than that. The first step in controlling your weight is to confront the problem honestly.

No particular diet is needed—just less of what you're having now. Cut out those elements in your present diet that are not particularly good for your body. Most of the "white" foods, such as breads and cakes, can easily be dispensed with. You want to keep fat intake as low as possible. You want at least five servings a day of foods high in fiber (whole grain breads, fruits, vegetables, salads, cereals). Your goal is to maintain a balanced diet with foods from each of the major groups.

A caution against fad diets: The statistics on long-term weight reduction from any of the current or past fads are discouraging. Basically, the individual depends on the fad rather than on making the more difficult long-term commitment to weight control. Almost any diet, maintained enthusiastically, will take some weight off. The liquid-protein diets appear dangerous; other diets, although generally safe, are not a permanent answer. If you use them, you must also make the long-term, permanent commitment to weight control.

Protect Your Joints

The first rule of joint protection is to listen to the pain messages your body sends and to do activities in the right way. Joints, ligaments, and bones can be damaged by misuse of a joint that is already inflamed or injured. Think of joint problems as being somewhat like a sprained ankle. The sprained ankle starts with an injury. There is pain and swelling, and it may hurt to walk. Your body is attempting to repair the sprained ligament; the repair takes place most rapidly if you are easy on the joint during the repair period. If you are too active you will sprain it again, and if you keep on spraining it you can have a long-term problem. On the other hand, you can't let a sprained ankle destroy your life, so you need to continue some activity. Listen to the pain message. If it hurts a lot, don't do it. If it is reasonably comfortable, go ahead. This is simply common sense—and that is the essence of joint protection.

Warm up your muscles and joints before activity. Stretch your body and your joints through all their motions. Slowly increase your activities, as would an athlete in training. Don't forget your common sense.

Some injuries, such as a torn meniscus or ligament in the knee, a broken hip, or a broken finger, can accelerate later development of arthritis. So avoiding activities likely to result in injury is another way of preventing arthritis. Football, baseball, and other activities that can result in injury do pose a hazard to the joints. Fractures resulting from falls in the elderly are a major problem and often could have been prevented. Minor tendinitis, stress fractures, and sprains may result from running or even walking; these do not lead to chronic arthritis.

In your exercise program, you are almost certain to develop some minor musculoskeletal problems. This doesn't mean the exercise is not good. It does mean you must use some restraint while exercising the injured part during its healing period.

Avoiding injury, listening to pain, wearing good shoes, maintaining good posture, and sleeping in a good bed are all methods of protecting the joints and preventing arthritis. In Part III we discuss the specific techniques for protecting individual joints and for solving common problems.

PART III

Solving Problems with Arthritis

Solutions

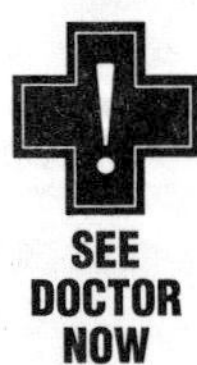

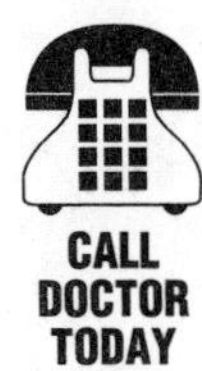

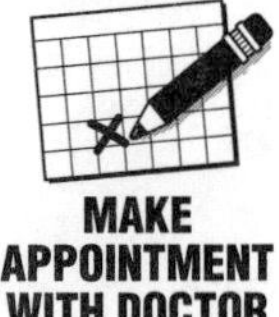

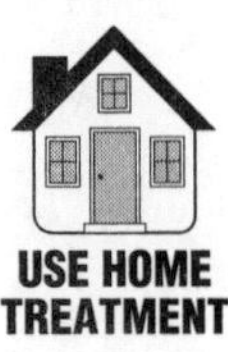

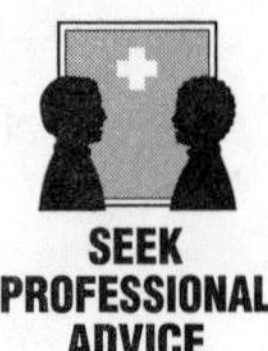

The discussions in this section relate to daily living. Arthritis can limit your everyday activities, for either the short term or the long term. These limitations are especially frustrating because we take our ability to perform simple everyday tasks for granted. The frustration sometimes leads to withdrawal rather than to confronting and dealing with the problems. Usually these problems are readily solved without professional help. Developing your own solutions can be a source of real satisfaction. If your arthritis is sufficiently severe to affect your daily life, take pride in finding ways to meet the challenge.

In the following 33 sections, common problems and their solutions are discussed using decision charts. Following the discussions of individual problems are two special sections, one on sexual problems and one on problems with employment. Look up your particular problems in the index or table of contents on the facing page. Then consult the appropriate pages to find your solutions. The decision charts will help you to decide whether to see the doctor. They also help you to know the urgency of your problem.

Sometimes the decision chart will tell you to "See Doctor Now." This indicates that an immediate visit to the doctor or emergency room is needed. More frequently it is better to "Call Doctor Today" for advice or to "Make Appointment with Doctor."

Much of the time you can take care of yourself using the "Home Treatment" suggestions in these sections. Remember that if home treatment does not work after a reasonable period, you should see the doctor.

Occasionally the book and decision charts recommend that you "Seek Professional Advice" by contacting an occupational therapist, physical therapist, counselor, etc. For certain problems, these professionals are better able to help you than a medical doctor.

Contents

SYMPTOM S1

1 Fatigue (Tiredness)

Most patients who have arthritis will experience some degree of fatigue. But most problems with fatigue are not physical weakness; they are related to depression, unhappiness, worry, or boredom. True weakness, with inability to move an arm or a leg, is a physical problem involving the nerves, brain, or muscle and needs immediate medical attention. Fatigue is far more common.

Another common cause of fatigue is overuse of one drug or another. Caffeine, leading to poor sleep habits, can cause daytime fatigue. Tranquilizers can make you feel tired or drowsy. Once the normal sleep cycle has been disturbed there is a tendency to grab an afternoon nap; then the following night's sleep is not good because the afternoon nap decreased the need for sleep at night. A vicious cycle has been set in motion.

You may be assuming from this discussion that most fatigue is not serious. That's correct. Even when arthritis is associated, most fatigue results from misunderstanding your body. Reestablishing a pattern of healthy activity, more moderate drug use, and good nocturnal sleep will do wonders.

But if your arthritis is an inflammatory one, such as rheumatoid arthritis or lupus, the disease may be causing the fatigue. This is a serious kind of fatigue and the measures above will not help much. In such cases the sed rate is elevated and there may be a low-grade fever. A hematocrit test may show the anemia of chronic disease. There may be some weight loss. Treatment of this kind of fatigue is based on treating the disease causing the fatigue; it may take some time to treat it correctly.

When you mention fatigue, most people don't even think of the problems listed above. They think of a problem with the thyroid, or of hypoglycemia, or of anemia. These are so unusual as causes of fatigue that you can almost forget about them. But if your fatigue persists more than six weeks despite home treatment, your doctor might want to check out these and other possibilities or may be able to reassure you that these problems are not present.

Fatigue is *not* old age. In fact, as you get older, you usually need less sleep and tend to be more alert, particularly early in the day. So pay attention to this symptom.

HOME TREATMENT

Listen to the fatigue message from your body. Heed it, but don't give in to it. Rest if you are tired, but alternate such periods with times of activity. Fatigue, because it can lead to physical deconditioning, can become its own cause.

Decrease all possible drugs, including caffeine, nicotine, alcohol, tranquilizers, and probably TV! Pep pills can cause fatigue, as can Valium and codeine. Suspect everything.

Increase new activities. Friends, hobbies, travel, vacations, and even shopping tend to break the fatigue cycle. Increase your activity level by addition of smooth, graded, and easy exercises. Exercise helps you become involved in new and different things, as well as giving physical help by increasing your stamina.

Expect improvement to be slow and expect to be discouraged at times. Persevere.

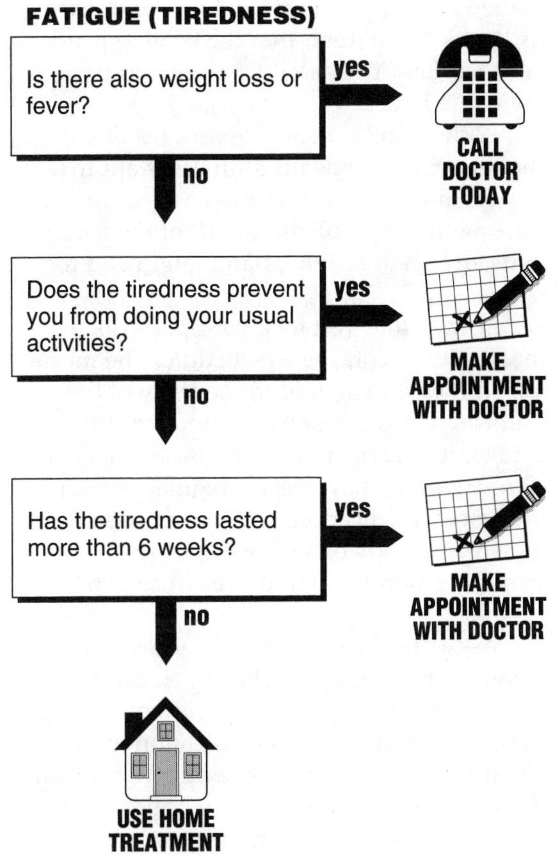

WHAT TO EXPECT AT THE DOCTOR'S OFFICE

The topics noted above will be explored in depth at the doctor's office, with particular attention to the drugs being taken and associated psychological events. The nerves and muscles will be the focus of the physical examination. Blood tests, including thyroid tests, hematocrit, sed rate, and others, may be ordered. Probably no abnormality will be found. If your doctor doesn't think that tests are necessary, don't insist.

Treatment will be essentially as above. The doctor will treat the fatigue by treating the disease underlying. Do not expect pep pills, tonics, vitamins, or other magic. And be patient.

SYMPTOM S2

2 Morning Stiffness

Morning stiffness is the hallmark of inflammatory rheumatic diseases. With a sprained ankle, with rheumatoid arthritis, with ankylosing spondylitis, or with other kinds of inflammation, you may notice that the sore area is stiff in the morning but loosens up as the day goes on. This phenomenon is most pronounced in rheumatoid arthritis and can be one of the patient's greatest aggravations.

No one really understands the reason for morning stiffness. Presumably, while the body is inactive, fluid leaks out from the small blood vessels and the tissues become waterlogged. Then if you try to move the part, the swollen tissues feel stiff until the motion pumps the fluid out through the lymph channels and the veins. If you sit or lie down during the day, the stiffness will return. This is called *gelling* or the *gel phenomenon,* after the behavior of gelatin, which remains liquid if kept moving and warm but solidifies if it sits for long. The phenomenon appears to be normal, but in the patient with inflammatory arthritis it can become a major problem.

Don't let morning stiffness keep you in bed. If your stiffness is that severe, call the doctor and discuss the problem today.

HOME TREATMENT

With a local condition, such as a sprained ankle or a tennis elbow, don't worry about the stiffness. Think of it as a normal part of the process of bringing healing materials to the injured area. Loosen up carefully before activity, and keep in mind that the healing is not yet complete. You should continue to protect the injured part.

With an inflammatory synovitis like rheumatoid arthritis the stiffness is apt to persist, and you are going to have to come to grips with the problem. Use all of the tricks you can to reduce the inflammation and the stiffness.

Be sure that you take your prescribed medication according to schedule. The morning stiffness is a sign of the severity of the arthritis, and the best way to reduce stiffness is to treat the arthritis. Your stiffness may be a signal that you have been irregular in taking prescribed medication. Or you may need more medication or a different drug. In particular, don't forget the last dose in the evening.

Ask your doctor about changing your medication schedule. Perhaps you can take a drug later in the evening or in the middle of the night so that there is medication in your blood in the morning when you are most stiff. If you are taking aspirin, some patients find that taking a coated aspirin (Ecotrin) immediately before retiring helps reduce the morning stiffness. These coated aspirin are absorbed more slowly, and the aspirin level lasts a bit longer. Avoid painkillers; they don't help morning stiffness.

Stretch gloves, of spandex or similar elastic material, may help morning stiffness of the hands if worn overnight. The idea is to prevent the tissues from becoming waterlogged. Give them a try. Take a warm bath or shower upon arising. Do gentle exercises. You will have a certain amount of stiffness each day, and you might as well get it worked out as soon as possible. Some people find that they are helped by using an electric blanket.

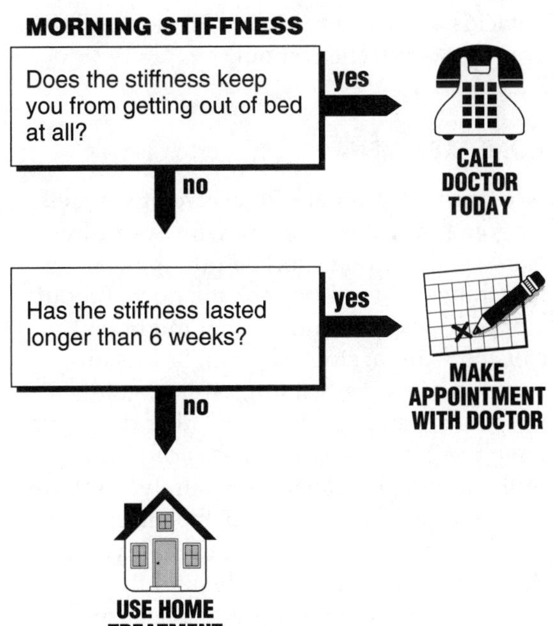

WHAT TO EXPECT AT THE DOCTOR'S OFFICE

The doctor's attention will be directed at control of the inflammation that is causing the stiffness. There may be an increase in your prescribed medication or a change to a different set of treatments. For example, gold and methotrexate are two agents that are often helpful. Formal physical therapy is not likely to help since the stiffness will have worked out by the time you reach the therapist. In inflammatory synovitis, increased morning stiffness is a signal for increased attention on the part of the doctor.

SYMPTOM S3

3 Weight Loss

Fortunately, weight loss is not very common with arthritis, but it is important when it occurs. A decline in weight that is not intentional and that results in falling below your ideal or normal weight is a signal that your body is not in equilibrium, that something substantial is wrong. Most people associate unwanted weight loss with cancer and may delay checking it out because they fear what might be found. This is not good thinking. Usually weight loss is a problem that can be helped; this is particularly true of weight loss associated with arthritis.

For example, weight loss may be a clue to depression. If you are a teenage girl or young woman, it may be *anorexia nervosa,* a psychiatric dysfunction that needs attention. It might be cancer, although usually not; if it is, early treatment is especially important. An overactive thyroid can cause loss of weight, as can an infection, serious but easily treated, like tuberculosis. With a connective-tissue disease, the arthritis condition can be causing the weight loss. Rheumatoid arthritis, polymyalgia rheumatica, lupus, polyarteritis, scleroderma, and polymyositis can all cause weight loss.

At any rate, weight loss is cause to see the doctor. An alarm bell has just rung. Check it out. It's hard to face the possibility of a major medical problem, but don't put it off.

Often a quite minor problem will be found. For example, difficulty in swallowing with scleroderma can result in weight loss and usually can be well treated. Or a drug may be upsetting the stomach, and some antacids and a change in medication will fix you up. Again, check it out.

HOME TREATMENT

Not much of that here. Take care of yourself by going over this problem with your physician. While getting checked out, there are a few things you can do. Ask the doctor about stopping any medications that might be causing nausea, stomach pain, or loss of appetite. Codeine, Valium, aspirin, gold injections, penicillamine, and other drugs may have these effects. If a drug has caused ulcers in the mouth, the doctor will surely want to stop it. If there is ulcerlike pain, antacids or cimetidine may be recommended. If you have the feeling of food sticking behind the breastbone, antacids may be used to decrease the irritation to your esophagus. And don't forget to cut down on alcohol and coffee (caffeine); these are two more drugs that are often overlooked.

WHAT TO EXPECT AT THE DOCTOR'S OFFICE

If depression is suspected, management will proceed as described in Depression **(S5).** If the cause is not clear, a careful evaluation will be forthcoming. Often this means a number of tests and may even mean hospitalization. If the weight loss could be related to arthritis, tests such as rheumatoid factor (latex) or serum-hepatitis antigen tests may be done. The thyroid may be checked. Chest X-ray, radiographs of the intestines, sigmoidoscopic examination (examination of the colon), and rectal examination may be needed. If you also have diarrhea, another set of tests are used to look for poor absorption of food. So expect some attention when you go to the doctor with this complaint.

WEIGHT LOSS

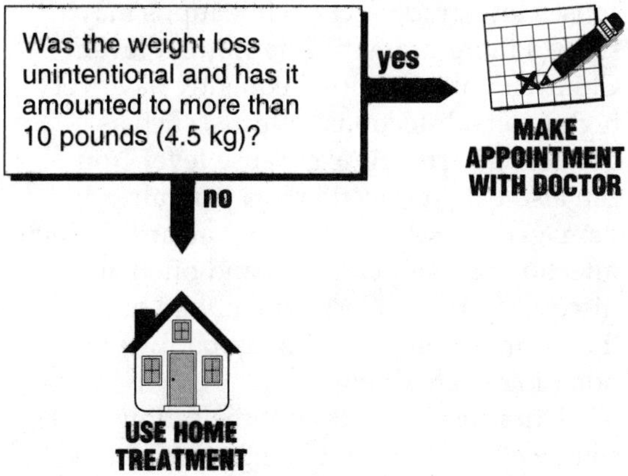

Was the weight loss unintentional and has it amounted to more than 10 pounds (4.5 kg)?

yes → **MAKE APPOINTMENT WITH DOCTOR**

no → **USE HOME TREATMENT**

SYMPTOM **S4**

4 Fever

Fever is not a disease; it is a symptom. It can mean anything or nothing, depending on its cause. In arthritis, fever can be a complicating infection in a joint or elsewhere, or it can be part of the disease, as in lupus, juvenile rheumatoid arthritis, or, more rarely, adult rheumatoid arthritis (RA). Of course, people with arthritis get fever for all the same reasons that anybody else does, and most fever with arthritis should not be treated any differently than if the person did not have arthritis. With fever, management is based on the condition that is causing the fever, not the fever itself.

Here are some points to keep in mind. Watch out for fever from a bacterial infection. This kind of fever requires the most urgent attention because antibiotics are necessary to treat the cause. Bacterial infections tend to be localized, and you usually can tell where the fever is coming from. It may be a sore throat, an earache, a boil, or a sore and swollen joint. Because of the way in which bacteria grow and divide, they are usually found in a single location, surrounded by pus cells—the body's response to the infection. With bacterial infections you may have a shaking chill. See the doctor if you suspect a bacterial infection. In contrast, viral infections tend to be less distinct; you may ache all over. These are less urgent, but any fever that persists for over a week should be checked out.

Arthritis-related fevers are few. Drug fever is the most common of these, and you should always start by suspecting your medication. Rheumatoid arthritis occasionally causes low-grade fever, while lupus may show a more dramatic intermittent fever. Children with arthritis frequently have very high fevers. Infectious arthritis, such as gonococcal arthritis, can cause fever. You can also get an infection in a joint already damaged by RA (or any other arthritis). Such infections are not common and often are discovered by an alert patient who notices that a single joint is acting up badly while other joints are doing well.

Duration separates out the serious fevers, so pay attention to how long your fever lasts, as noted on the decision chart opposite.

HOME TREATMENT

We discuss fever and its treatment in detail in *Take Care of Yourself* and *Taking Care of Your Child*, and you may want to refer to those books for more complete treatment of this subject. Here, with the assumption of an underlying arthritis, the same general principles hold.

You will usually be under the care of a doctor for your arthritis, and you may want to give your doctor a call to check out your plan for treating fever. If a drug might be causing the problem, ask about stopping the drug. If the fever might be related to the arthritis, you should see your doctor.

For flu, minor fevers from viral illnesses, and other problems, you can take acetaminophen in a dosage of 650 mg every four hours. For children, the appropriate dose is 65 mg every four hours for each year of age up to age ten, then the adult dose. Of course, if you are already taking aspirin for your arthritis, a call to the doctor is in order.

Keep the room cool. Wear light clothing. Children may require tepid baths to cool them

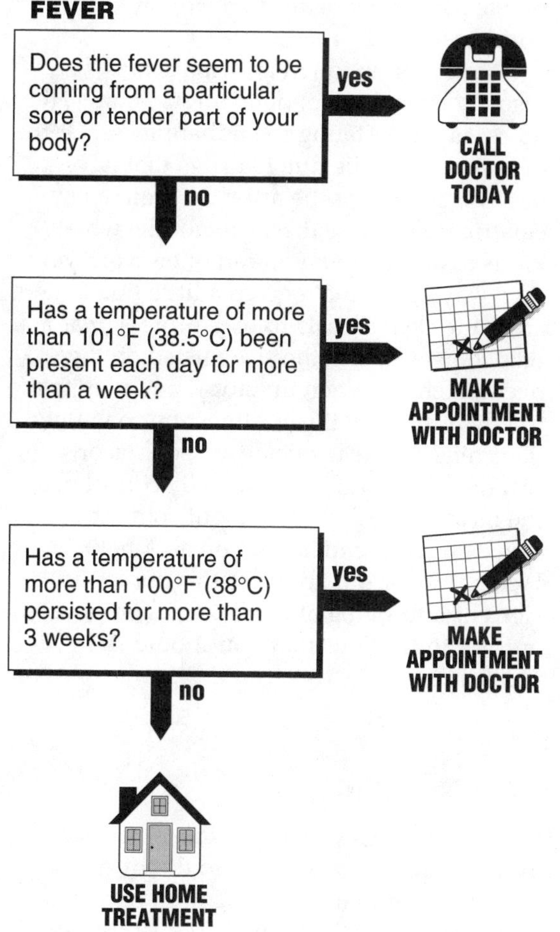

down. Regular use of these measures is better and more comfortable than allowing the fever to go up and down like a yo-yo.

WHAT TO EXPECT AT THE DOCTOR'S OFFICE

Examination and culture of any suspicious area for bacteria can be expected. A joint may be "tapped" and cultured. X-rays may be taken if a suspected infection is located near bone. Antibiotics may be prescribed if a bacterial infection is known or strongly suspected. Antibiotics do not help viral infections and should not be given for uncomplicated colds or flu.

SYMPTOM S5

5 Depression

Arthritis and depression are linked in the minds of many people. Perhaps this is because many of us associate arthritis with long-term pain, encroaching old age, or inevitability and hopelessness. Probably the general perception that "little can be done" for arthritis contributes to these feelings of futility.

In fact, most kinds of arthritis compare very favorably with other human ills. Consider loss of eyesight, loss of a limb, a stroke, diabetes, anginal heart pains, heart failure, or emphysema. Most patients with arthritis do not have as major a medical problem as patients with these illnesses. Further, much more can be done for the arthritis. So the hopelessness is mostly in our minds, and the reality is far better than our common perceptions.

All patients with arthritis can lead satisfying lives. Arthritis should not cause a prolonged reactive depression. A few weeks or months of adjustment are to be expected with severe arthritis, but things should and will get better.

With depression, there is hopelessness. Unhappy thoughts flood the brain, and you can't seem to shake them. You have trouble concentrating on anything for very long. You go to sleep all right but wake up early. Then you can't get back to sleep. Your speech and movements may be slow; your energy level is low. Your appetite is poor, and you may lose weight. You may be constipated. You may have aches and increased stiffness. All of these problems will get better as the depression improves.

Most depression in arthritis is *reactive* (usually overreactive) depression—that is, the illness is precipitating the unhappiness. Or the depression may be due to drugs that have been given to treat the arthritis. From a psychiatric standpoint, these are not the worst kinds of depression; you can often work your own way out of them given a little time. There are some clear signals to seek professional help, however, and these are listed on the decision chart. When unhappy, you may think briefly of suicide; this is almost normal. But if your reflections on suicide are serious or recurrent, or if you have actually considered the means by which you might commit suicide, it is essential that you seek help. Weight loss or unhappiness that shows no signs of improving after six weeks or more are also indications that you should see your physician.

HOME TREATMENT

Check the drugs you are taking. The easiest way to cure a depression is to discover and stop the drug that is causing it. In particular, worry about the "downers" frequently used as tranquilizers. These can cause depression. Valium, Librium, and similar drugs have little—perhaps no—place in the treatment of arthritis. Codeine and other painkillers can also cause depression or aggravate it. Antihistamines can do the same. Even sleeping medications, because of the unnatural type of sleep they induce, can contribute to depression. Some arthritis medications, notably prednisone and indomethacin, can cause depressive reactions. If you suspect any of these, call or visit the doctor.

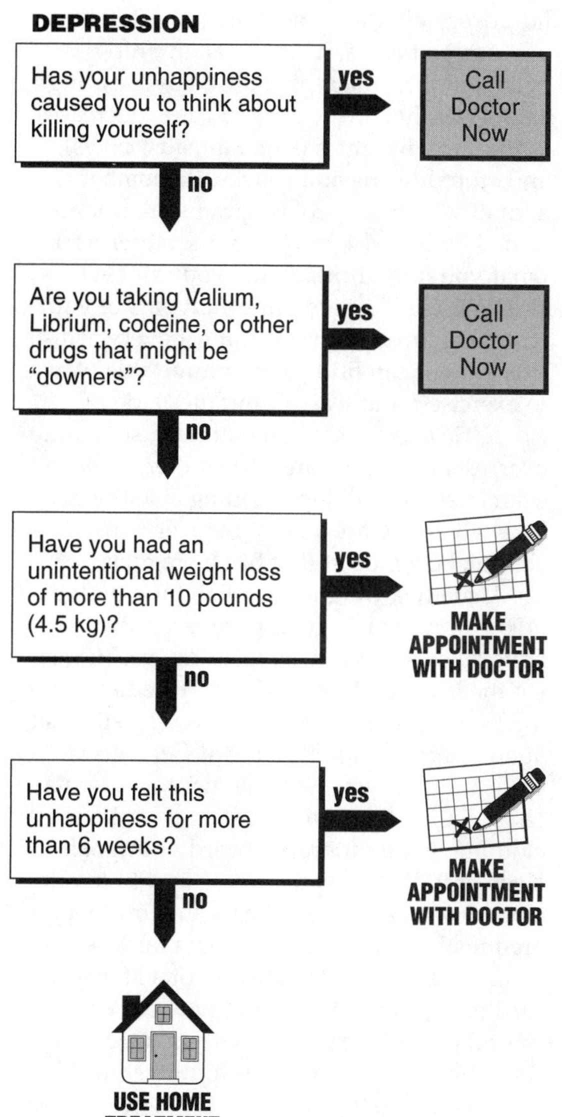

Increase activity and exercise. Friends, vacations, and new activities may need to be forced, but they will help lift the depression. Change your pace. Start new hobbies. Do things you've always wanted to do but kept putting off.

Project and anticipate future events. Find things to look forward to. Make long-range plans. Set intermediate goals. Work at living. Plan an exciting future event and begin saving and planning for it.

Know your limits. Get help when the signals are there. Most depressions ease if you work at life; a few don't and need some special care.

WHAT TO EXPECT AT THE DOCTOR'S OFFICE

A review of your medications and some changes, as well as discussion of the general factors mentioned above, can be expected. Sometimes blood tests, such as the hematocrit or thyroxine, will be ordered, although these usually are not helpful. Sometimes there may be referral to a psychiatrist or psychiatric social worker. Occasionally medications that fight depression may be prescribed. These antidepressant drugs can be very helpful but are not often required.

SYMPTOM **S6**

6 Overweight (Obesity)

Throughout this book, you've no doubt noticed the repeated emphais on the importance of weight control for managing your arthritis. Weight control is a difficult problem with no easy solutions. But it can be achieved. The principles of weight control are well established, and although you may not particularly enjoy it, you can successfully lose weight and keep it off.

First, check your diagnosis. Are you fat? Look at yourself naked in the mirror and be honest. Weight reduction and weight maintenance are life-and-death subjects; you can't afford to be dishonest with yourself or make jokes with your friends about your body weight. Fat shows, and the mirror is more accurate than the tables of "normal" weights and heights. Your answer may be that you are not fat. Great! Just watch your weight from time to time; don't talk or worry about a problem that you don't have.

HOME TREATMENT

There are two steps to your program: weight reduction and weight maintenance. You must continue the maintenance program for the rest of your life—that's the hard part. So much for "fast" diets; weight control goes on forever. Fortunately, weight maintenance is possible with over 95% of the calories that you would eat if you were fat and gaining. So while you need some privation, you do not need to starve yourself.

For weight reduction, almost any popular diet that is reasonably safe is all right. (Avoid liquid-protein diets; these are not safe.) Or you can just eat less. Don't eat anything between dinner and breakfast, have less high-calorie alcohol, decrease fat intake, decrease white carbohydrates (sugar, breads, cakes), and stop desserts and snacks. Remember that a lot of weight-control programs are undermined by impulse buying in the supermarket; what you don't bring home you can't eat.

Exercise is a very important part of your weight-control program. Almost every arthritis patient can find some comfortable way to exercise for at least 15 minutes a day: isometric exercises when you hurt, stretching exercises when you are stiff, and endurance exercises like walking or riding a stationary bike when you are able. Whatever you choose, be gentle at first but be regular.

Usually a weight loss of about a pound (450 g) a week is a good pace, even if you have 40 or 50 pounds to lose. You are in this for the long haul. Set early, intermediate, and long-term goals. Write them down. Tell others about them. Commit yourself! Get a good scale and plot your weight every week on a chart. Same day, same time, same scale, same clothing. Note progress toward your goal. Keep at it. Expect your rate of weight loss to slow down after a few days—the first pounds are mostly water and give you a false sense of progress anyway. Remember, total starvation results in a weight loss of only about one pound (450 g) a day, so any change greater than this simply represents a fluid shift that can reverse itself just as quickly. Over the long term, your graph will show your progress. Weight-loss groups, such as Weight Watchers, can be a big help.

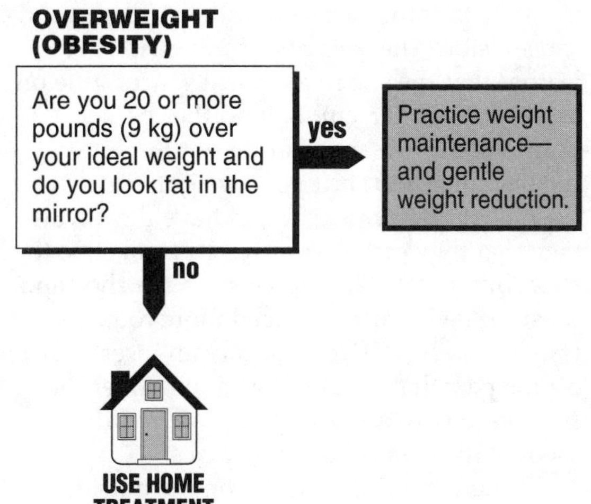

WHAT TO EXPECT AT THE DOCTOR'S OFFICE

Your doctor should give you the same advice that you have just read. Motivation and perseverance—not any magic treatments—are the keys to weight loss and maintenance. Pills are not useful for weight loss and can be hazardous. This is a home-treatment problem. Don't keep chasing rainbows; get to work.

SYMPTOM S7

7 Pain in the Ball of the Foot

The sole of your shoe wears at the "ball" of your foot, and your shoe may get a hole in it at that point. It wasn't true for our four-footed ancestors, but this is the point of greatest stress when we walk. We make it even worse by footwear designed for fashion rather than function. And unfortunately, this area is where the metatarsal bones join the toe bones; there are five important joints in each foot in this region. At these MTP, or metatarsalphalangeal, joints a great proportion of the arthritis that affects the foot occurs.

The consequences of arthritis in the forefoot (*metatarsalgia*) are minor yet adverse. With every step we place weight on this area, and it is difficult indeed to walk without using the forefoot. Even a small problem can make walking difficult, and other muscles, tendons, ligaments, and bones begin to lose strength. Serious attention by you is required because careful work at home can pay major dividends. Even though your arthritis is a systemic synovitis, you will find that attention to local factors can make all the difference.

Very rarely, you may have one of the indications on the decision chart to call your doctor. The questions in the chart are to make sure that you don't have gout, an infection, an unstable fracture, or nerve damage. Usually you won't, and this is then a home treatment problem.

HOME TREATMENT

The solution is usually quite simple. The principle is to move the weight bearing away from the painful part so that the inflammation can subside. The *metatarsal bar,* a strip of sole leather that the shoemaker will sew or glue on about an inch (2.5 cm) behind the contact point where you are wearing out the sole, is the key device to shift your weight. *Shoe inserts* help a few people and have the advantage that they can be transferred from shoe to shoe, but inserts take up room in the shoe and most toes with arthritis need more room rather than less. If you use a foam insert, cut off the part that would have gone under the sore place with scissors. You want to lift up the foot just behind the sore place.

The metatarsal bar goes on the outside. When you check your area of greatest pain against the area of greatest wear on the shoe, you will find that they are the same. Press on your foot about an inch (2.5 cm) behind the sore place and you will note how much better it feels and how the toes line up straighter. The metatarsal bar will also help your arch. It is an inexpensive device and any good shoemaker knows how to fit one. Fix several pairs of shoes.

Shoes are critical to problems of foot pain. Don't wear shoes with pointed toes. Avoid high heels—they throw additional weight on the forefoot. Look for a wide toe box. You can tell a lot in the store by walking around before buying; don't go home with a purchase that isn't comfortable, no matter what the salesperson says. Ask particularly to try the "Duckbill" made by the Joyce company or the "Roundabout" by Dr. Scholl. These shoes have a wide toe box and are comfortable for most; they are readily available, and they cost much less than specially made shoes. Try the athletic shoe department for casual shoes. The newer shoes designed for long-distance running on pavement are excellent for arthritis and should be more widely used; they are comfortable and less expensive than specially

PAIN IN THE BALL OF THE FOOT

Are any of these present?

- Unable to walk at all
- Fever
- Heat or redness at the area of pain
- Areas of numbness
- Significant injury
- Severe pain when *not* bearing weight
- Persistence after 6 weeks of home treatment

yes

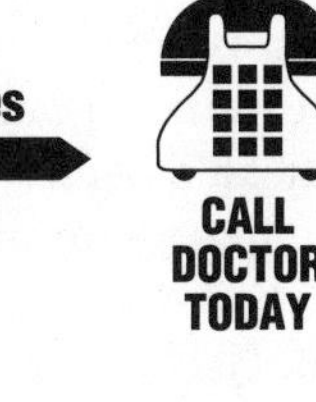

CALL DOCTOR TODAY

no

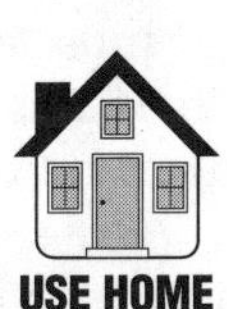

USE HOME TREATMENT

made shoes. Look for shoes with a good heel wedge support, a nylon upper that will spread in the toe box, and laces that run through guides rather than eyelets, so that they adjust smoothly. There are many good brands.

If your problem with pain in the forefoot occurs at night, you will need something to raise the covers off the foot. A pillow under the covers at the bottom of the bed is the easiest solution; a side-lying L-shaped piece of wood may be better for tall folks.

WHAT TO EXPECT AT THE DOCTOR'S OFFICE

The doctor will examine your foot and ankle and sometimes take an X-ray. Advice will be much the same as that given above. Injection is occasionally of some use. Fancy shoes may be ordered, but if you have followed the instructions under Home Treatment you are likely to be disappointed when the $400 shoes aren't as comfortable as those selected in a shoestore. If problems are persistent surgery is sometimes required and is often well worthwhile. Bunionectomy, metatarsal head resection, and resection of a Morton's neuroma (tumor) are three frequently useful procedures. The operation for putting plastic joints in the forefoot is not yet perfected. Finally, your doctor may increase anti-inflammatory medications to improve the underlying arthritis.

SYMPTOM S8

8 Heel Pain

Heel pain can occur at one of two places: the bottom of the heel or the back of the heel. The heel bone, the calcaneus, is the largest bone of the foot and bears our full weight during part of each stride. The painful heel, in almost all instances, is caused by excessive strain on one of the two major ligaments, and the pain occurs where these ligaments attach. The Achilles tendon attaches at the back of the heel. This is the strongest tendon in the body and connects the muscles on the back of the calf to the heel. The force of contraction of the muscles enables us to stand on tiptoe and gives an extra thrust as we walk or run. Damage to this tendon attachment is called Achilles tendinitis. Frequently there will also be tears in the tendon itself or in the lower part of the muscle.

The heel-spur syndrome affects the bottom of the heel. This is where the ligaments that make up the arch of the foot attach to the heel bone. These ligaments function like a bowstring to arch the foot, so you can see that they are under pressure every time we stand or step. If the problem persists, calcium may develop in the inflamed area where the ligaments attach. The presence of the calcium spur may or may not cause additional pain; often the spur itself is the only visible part of a painful process. Many people have pain without visible spurs, while others have spurs but no pain.

Heel pain of both back and bottom type can occur in Reiter's syndrome or ankylosing spondylitis. Here the process is the same except that no injury is required and rest is not as effective a treatment. Even more rarely, gout or infection will be present. Usually heel pain is the simple result of a forgotten injury.

HOME TREATMENT

Rest, avoidance of further injury, and gradual resumption of activity as the pain subsides are indicated. Activities not requiring weight bearing, like swimming, can be continued full tilt.

For Achilles tendinitis, rest the foot or feet. Use a shoe with a high heel wedge and a lot of padding, since this limits the stretch on the tendon. Warm up carefully for ten or fifteen minutes before activities that might cause reinjury, and avoid sudden starts, particularly on cold days. Tennis and running uphill are not good. Remember that tight muscles on the back of the leg put extra strain on this tendon, so warm up with toe-touching or hurdler-position exercises.

For the heel-spur syndrome, activities to avoid are ones that flatten the foot and put strain on the bowstring.

The best treatment is to tightly strap the foot just ahead of the front of the heel and

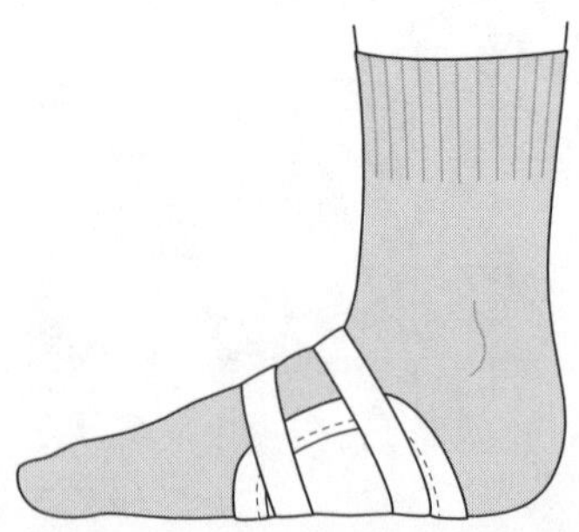

Heel pain relief. When properly positioned, a strap like the one shown will give immediate relief. If your foot hurts, swells, or becomes cold, the strap is too tight. The strap may be worn with or without a sock.

HEEL PAIN

Are any of these present?
- Unable to walk at all
- Fever
- Areas of numbness
- Heat or redness in the area of pain
- Severe pain when *not* bearing weight
- Persistence after 6 weeks of home treatment

yes

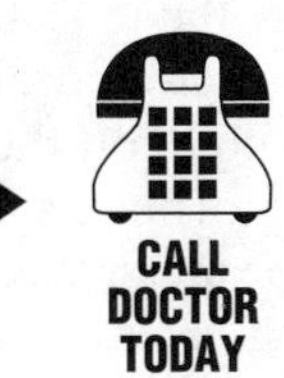

CALL DOCTOR TODAY

no

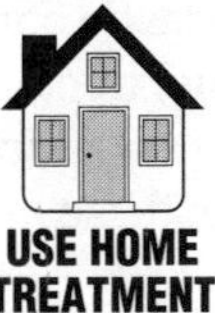

USE HOME TREATMENT

relieve the stress on the ligament; the stress will be taken by the strap. You can use a "tennis elbow" strap or purchase a "heel pain" Velcro device. Do not cut off the circulation by making the strap too tight; the foot should not hurt or become cold. (A second shoelace laced through the top two eyelets and tightened also may work.) If you get it right, the pain on walking will go away immediately. Healing takes six weeks, however.

After six weeks of treatment, check with your doctor if you are still having trouble.

WHAT TO EXPECT AT THE DOCTOR'S OFFICE

Your doctor will examine the painful areas and give you advice like that above. If Reiter's syndrome or ankylosing spondylitis is present, major relief may be obtained from indomethacin or other nonsteroidal anti-inflammatory agents. These drugs should not be used for injuries as a rule since they suppress the healing inflammatory response. Injection of steroids into the Achilles tendon area is quite dangerous and should be avoided; the entire tendon will sometimes rip apart after an injection has weakened it.

SYMPTOM S9

9 Ankle Pain

The ankle is a large joint, with lots of synovium to get inflamed. Since it is a weight-bearing joint it is unavoidably stressed at each step. As a result, synovitis is usually not the direct cause of pain or instability of the ankle joint. Most frequently, the problem is in the ligaments near the joint. The sprained ankle is a simple example of this. With an ankle sprain, the ligament attaching the bump on the outer side of the ankle to the outer surface of the foot is injured at one or both ends. The ankle itself is all right. With rheumatoid arthritis the synovitis may have injured the adjacent ligaments so that the joint slips, ligaments are strained, and pain and instability result. Walking on an unstable joint just increases the damage, but if you can stabilize the joint walking is usually all right.

If you look down your leg when lying and when standing, you can tell if the joint is stable. If it is unstable, the line of weight going down your leg will not be straight down the foot. Perhaps the foot will be slipped a half inch or an inch (1.3 or 2.5 cm) to the outside of where it should be. When you are not bearing weight, it will move back in line toward a more normal position. The unstable joint may actually slip sideways if you try to move the foot with your hands.

Rarely, infection or gout may be the cause of this problem; the questions on the decision chart are designed to minimize this possibility.

HOME TREATMENT

Listen to the pain message; it is telling you to rest the part a bit more, to provide support for the unstable ankle, to back off on your exercise progression, or to use an aid to take weight off the ankle.

The unstable ankle should be supported for major weight-bearing activity. Instability is not just a swollen ankle; the ankle must be displaced sideways or be crooked. Support is most simply obtained by high-lacing boots, but sometimes these will be too uncomfortable and you will have to have specially made boots or an ankle brace. Professional help is required for adequate fitting of such devices.

For the stable ankle, an elastic bandage and a shoe with a comfortable, thick heel pad will help. You should select a "walking" shoe that goes up above the ankle; these are available at athletic shoe stores.

Crutches are often a big help for a flare-up, and even a cane can help you take weight off the sore ankle. Remember to have the crutches short enough so as not to injure the nerves in your armpits. When you use the crutches, take the weight on your hands or arms.

If you have a synovitis, then make sure that you have been taking your medication exactly as prescribed. Sometimes a patient gets a little bored and lax with the pill-taking routine and, a few days later, experiences difficulty walking because of pain or swelling.

As soon as the pain begins to decrease, you can gently begin to exercise the joint again. Swimming is good because you don't have to bear weight. Start easy and slow with your exercises. Sit on a chair, let the leg hang free, and wiggle the foot up and down and in and out. Later, walk carefully with an ankle bandage for support. Stretch the ankle by

ANKLE PAIN

Are any of these present?

- Unable to walk at all
- Fever
- Severe pain when *not* bearing weight
- Heat and redness in the area of pain
- Persistence after 6 weeks of home treatment

yes → CALL DOCTOR TODAY

no ↓

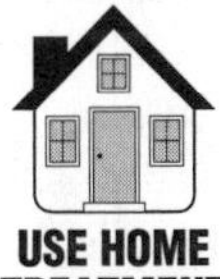

USE HOME TREATMENT

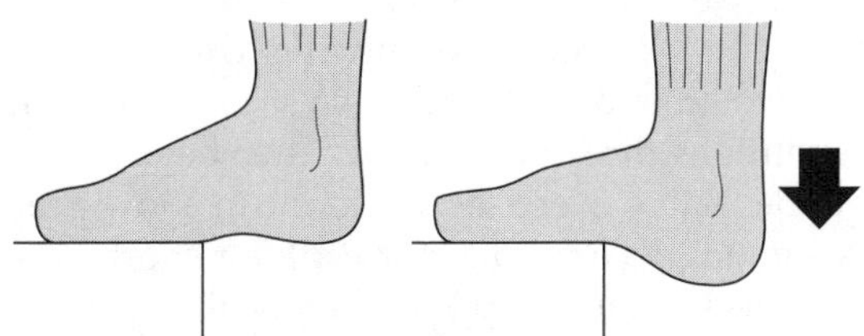

putting the forefoot on a step and lowering the heel. As the ankle gains strength, you can walk on tiptoe and walk on your heels to stretch and strengthen the joint. Do the exercises several times a day; the ankle shouldn't be a lot worse after the exercise if you aren't overdoing it. Keep at it, but take your time.

WHAT TO EXPECT AT THE DOCTOR'S OFFICE

The doctor will examine the painful area and may take X-rays. The dose of anti-inflammatory drugs may be increased. Special shoes or braces may be prescribed. Surgery is occasionally necessary. Fusion (nonmotion) of the ankle is the most generally useful procedure; a fixed, pain-free ankle is often preferable to an unstable and painful one. The artificial ankle joint is not yet satisfactory for most people, but progress is rapid in this area.

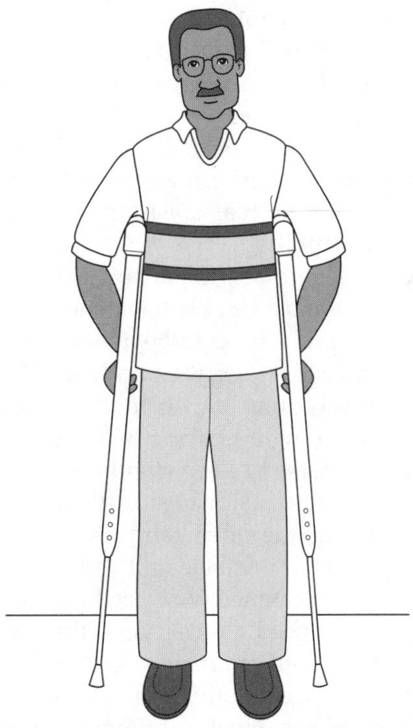

Crutches. When you stand straight, the crutches should reach from six inches to the side of each foot to two inches (three or four fingers' width) below the armpits. Take the weight on your hands.

SYMPTOM S10

10 Knee Pain

The knee is a hinge. It is, of course, a large, weight-bearing joint. But it is a hinge, and its motion is much more strictly limited than that of most other joints. It will straighten to make the leg a stable support and it will bend (flex) to more than a right angle. However, it cannot move in any other direction. The limited motion of the knee gives it great strength, but it is not engineered to take side stresses, as football players discover each year.

There are two cartilage compartments in each knee—one inner and one outer. If the cartilage wears unevenly, the leg can bow in or out. Or if you are born with crooked legs, there can be strain that causes the cartilage to wear more rapidly.

To work normally the knee must be stable, and it must be able to extend fully to a straight leg. If it lacks full extension, the muscles have to support the body at all times and strain is continuous; normally our knee "locks" in a straight position and allows us to rest (or a horse to sleep standing up). If the knee wobbles from side to side, there is too much stress on the side ligaments.

If the knee is unstable and wobbles or if it cannot be straightened, you need the doctor. Similarly, you need a physician if there is a possibility of gout or an infection; the knee is the joint most frequently bothered by these serious problems. Finally, if there is pain or swelling in the calf below the sore knee, you may have a blood clot, but more likely you have a *Baker cyst* and you need the doctor. These cysts start as fluid-filled sacs in an inflamed knee but enlarge through the tissues of the calf and may cause swelling quite a distance below the knee.

HOME TREATMENT

Listen to the pain message and try not to do things that aggravate the pain either immediately or the next day. If there has been a recent injury, then an elastic bandage may help; otherwise, probably not. Use of a cane can help; the cane is best carried in the hand on the side of the painful knee by some, while others carry it on the opposite side.

Do *not* use a pillow under the knee at night or at any other time as this can make the knee stiffen so that it cannot be straightened.

Exercises should be started slowly and performed several times daily if possible. Swimming is good because there is no weight-bearing requirement. From the beginning, pay close attention to flexing and straightening the leg. A friend can help, since it may be more comfortable to move the leg passively. But work at getting it straight and keeping it straight. Next, begin isometric exercises. Tense the muscles in your upper leg, front and back at the same time, so that you are exerting force but your leg is not moving. Exert force for two seconds, then rest two seconds. Do ten repetitions three times a day. Then begin gentle, active exercises. A bicycle in a low gear is a good place to start. Or walk for short distances. *Avoid* deep knee bends; they place too much stress on the knee.

Knee problems can come from the feet, as from jogging or tennis. Wearing comfortable shoes with good support and a lot of padding can help your knees; many people get relief from use of good "running shoes," which are designed to minimize impact.

Make sure that you are taking your medication as directed, since your painful knee could be caused by too little medication.

KNEE PAIN

Are any of these present?

- Unable to walk at all
- Rapid development of swelling without injury
- Fever
- Recent injury, and knee wobbles from side to side or can't be straightened
- Severe pain when *not* bearing weight
- Pain and swelling in calf below swollen knee
- Persistence after 6 weeks of home treatment

yes

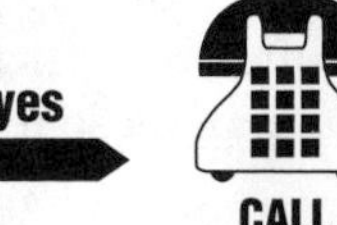

CALL DOCTOR TODAY

no

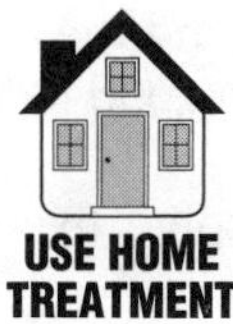

USE HOME TREATMENT

WHAT TO EXPECT AT THE DOCTOR'S OFFICE

The doctor will examine the knee and other joints, and possibly X-ray the knee. If a Baker cyst is suspected, or for diagnostic reasons, some fluid may be drawn from the knee through a needle and tested. This procedure is easy, not too uncomfortable, and quite safe. If you have an unstable knee after an injury, you may need surgery to repair the torn ligaments or remove the torn cartilage. If you have synovitis, a synovectomy (removal of the synovium) may be recommended. This can be useful, but it is an operation about which you may want to get a second opinion. For severe problems, total knee replacement may be recommended. This is a good operation and often gives total pain relief. Other operations include removal of bits of bone or cartilage (joint mice), and removal of some bone (osteotomy) in order to straighten the leg. Arthroscopic surgery is increasingly used, and recovery is much faster after this more minor procedure.

SYMPTOM S11

11 Hip Pain

The hip is a "ball-and-socket" joint. The largest bone in the body, the femur, is in the thigh, and narrows to a neck that angles into the pelvis and ends in a ball-shaped knob. This ball fits into a curved socket in the pelvic bone (acetabulum). This arrangement provides a joint that can move freely in all directions. The joint itself is located rather deeply under some big muscles so that it is protected from dislocating—that is, from coming out of the socket.

Two problems arise because of this arrangement of the anatomy. The neck of the femur can break rather easily, and this is usually what happens when an older person "breaks a hip" after a slight fall. Also, the "ball" part of the joint must get its blood supply from below, and the small artery that supplies the "head" of the femur can get clogged, leading to death of the bone and a kind of hip arthritis called *aseptic necrosis.*

The hip joint can also get infected, and rarely, it will be the site for an attack of gout. The bursae that lie over the joint can be inflamed with a bursitis. True synovitis, as in rheumatoid arthritis, can injure the joint. And it is not uncommon for attachment arthritis, such as ankylosing spondylitis, to cause stiffness or loss of motion at the hip.

A *flexion contracture* means that motion at the hip joint has been partly lost. The hip becomes partially fixed in a slightly bent position. This causes the pelvis to tilt forward, so that when you walk or stand straight, the back has to curve a little extra. This throws strain on the low back area.

For poorly understood reasons, pain in the hip is often felt down the leg, often at the knee or just above. This is called *referred pain.* Nonreferred hip pain may be felt in the groin or the upper, outer thigh. Pain that starts in the low back is often felt in the region of the hip. Since the hip joint is so deeply located, it can often be difficult to locate the exact source of pain in these regions.

HOME TREATMENT

Listen for the pain message and try to avoid activities that are painful or aggravate pain. You will want to avoid pain medication as much as possible. Rest the joint from painful activities. Use a cane or crutches if necessary. The cane is usually best held in the hand *opposite* the painful hip since this allows greater relaxation in the large muscles around the hip joint. Move the cane and the affected side simultaneously, then the good side, then repeat.

As the pain begins to resolve, exercise should be gradually introduced. First, use gentle motion exercises to free the hip and prevent stiffness. Stand with your good hip by a table and lean on the table with your hand. Let the bad hip swing front and back and side to side. Lie on your back with your body half off the bed and the bad hip hanging, and let the leg stretch backward toward the floor. See how far apart you can straddle your legs, and bend the upper body from side to side. Try to turn your feet apart like Charlie Chaplin, so that the rotation ligaments get stretched. Repeat these exercises three times a day.

Then introduce more active exercises to strengthen the muscles around the hips. Lie on your back and raise your legs one at a time. You can bend the other leg at the knee if it feels better. Repeat three times for each leg; build up to ten repetitions.

HIP PAIN

Are any of these present?

- Inability to walk at all
- Fever
- Severe pain when *not* bearing weight
- Recent injury
- Persistence after 6 weeks of home treatment

yes → **CALL DOCTOR TODAY**

no → **USE HOME TREATMENT**

Swimming stretches muscles and builds good muscle tone. Bicycle or walk. When walking, start with short strides and gradually lengthen them as you loosen up. Gradually increase your effort and distance, but not by more than 10% each day. A good firm bed can help, and the best sleeping position is on your back. Avoid pillows beneath the knees or under the low back.

WHAT TO EXPECT AT THE DOCTOR'S OFFICE

Expect examination of the hip and motion of the hip, as well as your other joints and your back. X-rays may be taken. Anti-inflammatory medication may be increased. Unfortunately, there is some evidence that too much anti-inflammatory medication can accelerate the progression of the arthritis. Injection is only rarely used or needed. One of several surgical procedures may be recommended if the pain is bad and persistent or if you are having real problems walking. Total hip replacement, a remarkable operation, has largely superseded many older techniques. It is almost always successful in stopping pain and may help mobility a great deal. The artificial hip should last at least ten or fifteen years with current techniques. You get up and around quite quickly after surgery, and the complications are rather rare. Other procedures include pinning the hip, replacing either the ball or the socket, but not both, or removing a wedge of bone to straighten out the joint angle.

Hip exercise. Lying on your back with your body half off the bed, let the bad hip hang, and let the leg stretch backward toward the floor.

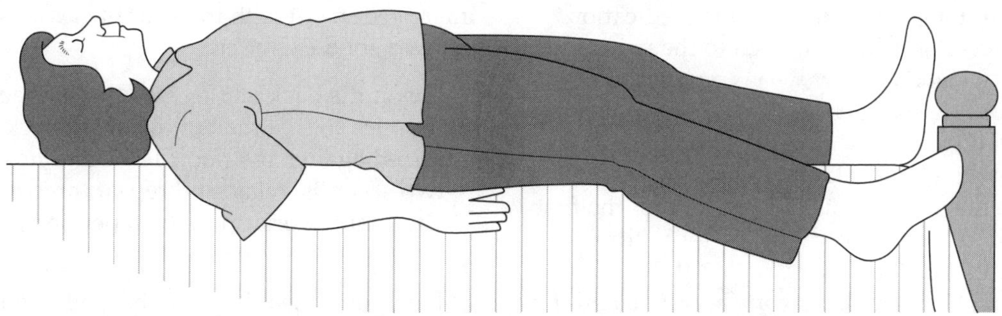

SYMPTOM S12

12 Low Back Pain

Low back pain—practically a universal problem—is discussed on pages 76–81. The crucial things to remember are that this problem is common (most people get it), painful (incredibly), medically minor (most of the time), and that the cause is nearly always an injury that requires time to heal completely. You may or may not have noticed the injury. Medication cannot speed the healing process. If there is any sign of nerve damage, or if a fracture might have occurred, or if the pain just won't go away, see the doctor.

HOME TREATMENT

Think of a sprained ankle. The injury causes bruising and swelling for two or three days, then slow healing begins. Pain is better in less than a week, but six weeks is required for full healing. Reinjury means that the healing process must start again from the beginning. Low back pain is the same.

Do *not* take all kinds of painkillers and muscle relaxants and then go on as if your back were all right; this practice will likely lead to reinjury. Either take the medication and rest flat in bed, or listen to the pain message and do only what you can do in reasonable comfort.

Don't apply heat to the area the first day; if anything, use cold packs to decrease pain. Heat may be cautiously applied after the first day, but it really won't help a lot. A firm mattress or a bed board is part of the standard advice; back problems vary, however, and if you are more comfortable at night and the following morning with a slightly softer mattress, use that. Aspirin or other mild pain relievers are probably all right, but they won't help much. A small pillow or folded towel beneath the low back may increase your comfort when sleeping flat. When you get up, draw your knees up, then roll sideways and sit up. The position of lying on your side, knees up, is more comfortable than lying on the back for many people.

You doubtless have muscle spasms. Although painful, they are protecting your injured back. If you can last out the discomfort without muscle relaxants and without a lot of pain medication, your back may heal more strongly and you decrease the chance of reinjury.

Exercises shouldn't be started for a week or so until things feel a lot better, and then they should be begun slowly. Exercise is designed to make recurrence less likely by toning the muscles and ligaments so that the spine has greater strength. Abdominal muscles assist spinal stability and are part of the exercise program. If you have some weight to lose, get started with the weight reduction right away.

Exercises should be repeated several times daily and gradually increased in number and in effort expended. Toe-touching, side-bending, and twisting exercises are *not* particularly good; for the back, you are more interested in strength than suppleness. Here are two good exercises:

1. Lie on the back and tighten the stomach muscles so that the hollow of the back is forced against the floor. Tense and hold for two seconds, relax, and repeat three times. Gradually work up to ten repetitions.

2. Lie on your back, pillow under your head. Hug your knees to your chest with your

LOW BACK PAIN

Are any of these present?

- Weakness or numbness in one or both legs
- Pain going down a leg below the knee
- Significant fall or injury
- Fever without flulike aches
- Persistence after 6 weeks of home treatment

yes → **CALL DOCTOR TODAY**

no ↓

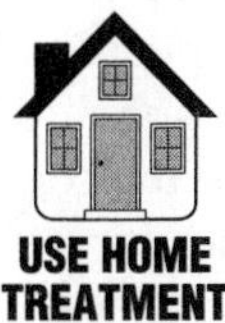

USE HOME TREATMENT

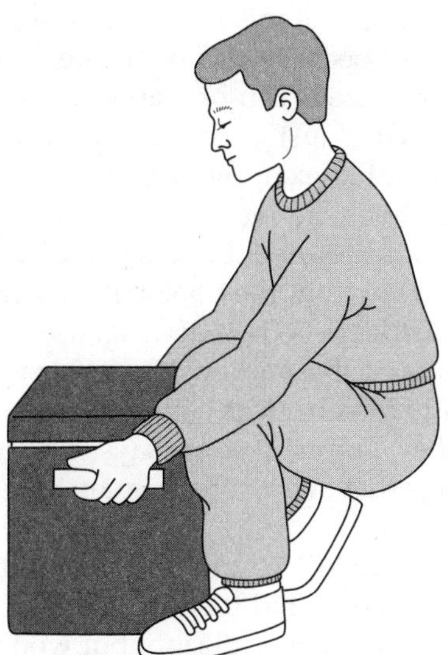

Lifting heavy objects. To avoid back strain, bend your knees, keeping your back straight and erect.

hands, exhale so that your spine can curve as much as possible, hold for five seconds, relax, and repeat three times. Work up to ten repetitions.

Posture helps. Sit in a straight chair. Keep your shoulders back. Have a good mattress on your bed. Lift weight with your legs, not your back. Never lift from a bending forward position. Avoid sudden shifts and strains, particularly those that throw the upper body backwards. Tennis, for example, should not be rushed as your back recovers. You can safely walk, swim, or bicycle long before it would be safe to resume your tennis game. The best book for self-management of back pain is *Good News for Bad Backs,* listed in Appendix B.

WHAT TO EXPECT AT THE DOCTOR'S OFFICE

Don't expect much. Unless there is nerve injury, the doctor doesn't have much to offer. Surgery is best reserved for patients with nerve-compression syndromes or for particularly severe and persistent difficulties. Failure of surgery to improve back problems is rather common.

The commonly used drug regimens of painkillers and muscle relaxants have never been shown to shorten recovery or to help prevent recurrence; under some circumstances these drugs can increase the chance of reinjury and can thereby delay healing. These drugs also affect your thinking processes and offer some hazard if you drive a car or operate heavy machinery. Uncomplicated low back strain is a problem for home treatment first.

If there is nerve injury, traction or surgery can help, and your delay in seeking medical care could have permanent consequences. So keep looking for the danger signs of weakness, numbness, or pain going down the leg below the knee.

SYMPTOM S13

13 Neck Pain

Someone who is a "pain in the neck" just keeps bothering you and won't go away. Neck pain is thus so memorable that it has reference in folk idiom. Most people have neck pain at some point, and occasionally a person has quite serious problems.

The neck bones are a continuation of the spine. The top seven vertebrae are called *cervical* or *neck vertebrae.* The seventh one makes the prominent bump you can feel where your back joins your neck. The uppermost vertebra, the atlas, holds up the skull. The second vertebra, the axis, has a vertical peg (odontoid), around which the head turns. The entire neck is more flexible than the back; it bears less weight but is less well protected by thick muscles. The disk spaces in the neck can get narrow, bony spurs can form, and nerves can get caught and compressed, just as in the low back. Spondylitis and other forms of attachment arthritis can affect the neck, and rheumatoid arthritis is particularly likely to affect the top two vertebrae, allowing the head to slip forward and backward on the neck. Injuries to the ligaments of the neck take some time to heal.

Usually, like a low back problem, a neck problem is minor and will be self-limited. It must depend on natural healing processes to resolve. Excessive neck movement tends to slow the healing and has the possibility of causing reinjury.

HOME TREATMENT

Rest the neck and listen for what the pain message tells you not to do. You can take a bath towel, fold it lengthwise so that it is a four-inch-wide (10 cm) strip, and wrap the neck with it, securing it comfortably with a safety pin or tape. Now you have a soft neck brace to wear at night, and this will clear up nearly half of all neck pain problems. If things persist, use the soft collar during the day as well, or buy a commercial soft collar to wear. You want some support from the collar, but more than that you want a little reminder not to turn your head too fast or too far.

If you have pain going down toward your shoulders, you may have some nerve compression. Here the best neck position is flexed forward about 15 degrees to open up the channels for the nerves. Take the cover off of your neck collar and trim the chin spot about one-half inch (1.3 cm), then replace. Use a wide (usually 4-inch [10 cm]) collar.

Watching a tennis match is obviously not a good idea because of the repeated head turning required. You probably engage in other activities just as damaging without realizing it. For example, wearing your glasses while reading may decrease the neck movements required, because you will be farther away from the book. Sit back farther from your work. When driving, use the mirrors carefully, and avoid turning your neck around to look back. A collar will help you remember. Common sense says to watch out for things that aggravate the pain and to stop doing them.

Keep painkillers and muscle relaxants to a minimum or avoid them altogether. Aspirin or acetaminophen is all right but won't make you feel much better. Sleep on a good firm mattress. Don't sleep on your stomach, and

NECK PAIN

Are any of these present?

- Numbness, tingling, or pain shooting up over the scalp
- Significant fall or injury
- Fever without flulike aches
- Weakness or numbness in the arms or legs
- Persistence after 6 weeks of home treatment

yes

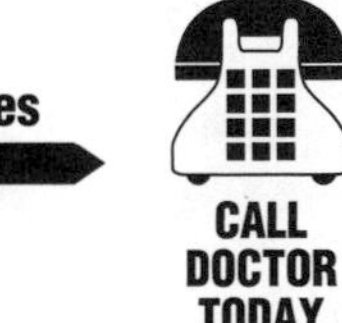

CALL DOCTOR TODAY

no

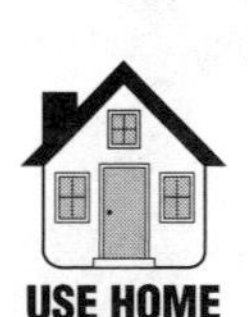

USE HOME TREATMENT

if you sleep on your side, place a pillow so that your neck is in a neutral position, not propped up or hanging down. When lying on your back, place the pillow beneath your neck as well as your head. The pillow should be a small one. You can buy pillows with side wings, which help stabilize the neck; look for those designed for airplane use, available in travel stores. Don't reach or look over your head to get objects; use a stool.

Exercises begin as the pain subsides, usually after five to seven days. Don't rush them—they are designed to help prevent the next recurrence. There are two types of exercises, the stretching exercises and the strengthening exercises, and you should do some of each.

Start stretching exercises with gentle stretches, and increase the stretch slowly day by day. Do them twice daily, each maneuver three times. There are three exercises: chin toward chest, ear toward shoulder, and look to the side. The last two should of course be done in each direction.

Strengthening exercises can begin at the same time, and start with three repetitions twice daily. Slowly work up to ten repetitions. If you have been having recurrent neck problems, the exercises are a worthwhile lifetime habit. Here are three:

- Raise both shoulders toward ears, hold for two seconds, relax, repeat.
- Take a deep, deep breath, hold for five seconds, release, repeat. The neck muscles are "accessory muscles of respiration," and breathing exercises involve the neck.
- While standing with both hands behind your back, grab one thumb with your other hand. Flex your head way back. Press down with your hand. Take a deep breath,

relax, repeat. This exercise can be done lying on your stomach as well, after you get good at it standing up.

A hot shower may increase comfort while exercising. Some authorities recommend doing the exercises in the shower.

WHAT TO EXPECT AT THE DOCTOR'S OFFICE

The uncomplicated neck pain problem is a job for home treatment. If there is pressure on a nerve, then hospitalization, traction, myelograms, CT or MR scans, or surgery may be needed. But if there is no nerve pressure the doctor has relatively little additional advice to offer. Surgery in the neck is inconsistent in relieving the problem. If your long-term neck problem doesn't have any "objective" findings and X-rays don't reveal a physical problem, a visit to a psychiatrist may be recommended. Tension headaches are a simple emotional problem that can localize in the neck muscles. Similarly, other psychiatric syndromes sometimes underlie a pain in the neck that just won't go away.

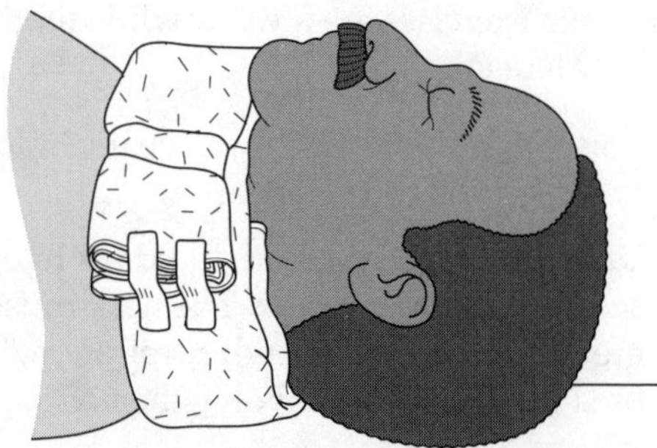

Neck pain relief. An ordinary bath towel, wrapped around the neck at bedtime, may alleviate some neck pain caused by poor sleeping habits.

SYMPTOM **S14**

14 Shoulder Pain

When the shoulder is affected by a problem it has a tendency to become "frozen," regardless of the nature of the problem. The frozen shoulder is stiff, limited in motion, and can be permanent if not appropriately treated. Understanding the way the shoulder works will help you understand the many different injuries that result in the same general problem.

The shoulder is our largest non-weight-bearing joint and has a complicated set of motions. Actually, the motions come from a series of three different joints that, in combination, give us the ability to swing our arms every which way, together with reasonable strength and stability at the joint.

If you lift your arm straight up over your head, you can feel the three joints come into play one after the other by using your other hand to feel the movement of the bones. The first 90 degrees of motion, from arm-at-the-side to arm-straight-out-to-the-side, come from the true shoulder joint. This joint is a shallow ball and socket held together by a tough fibrous capsule, lined with synovial cells and covered with tendons and muscles. It connects the arm to the shoulder blade.

As you raise your arm higher the shoulder blade begins to move, because of motion at a fibrous joint that joins the shoulder blade to the collarbone. This allows perhaps 75 degrees more of motion. Finally, the entire collarbone begins to tilt up, moving at a fibrous joint connecting the collarbone to the breastbone. This intricate design permits more motion at the shoulder joint than at any other joint.

An injury of any kind tends to immobilize this complex apparatus, and the inflammation that is helping repair the damage can involve nearby tissues. As healing occurs, adhesions may stick surfaces together and motion can be lost—hence, the frozen shoulder. This stiffening process is much more common in the shoulder than in any other joint.

The causes can be many: athletic injury, calcific tendinitis, rheumatoid arthritis, aseptic necrosis, ankylosing spondylitis, and many other conditions that start either in the joint itself or in the bursae or the surrounding ligaments. Much more rarely, gout, pseudogout, or infection can be present.

The decision chart indicates that you won't have to see the doctor for most shoulder problems. However, be rather careful with the shoulder. If your home treatment is not progressing well, don't put off the doctor visit too long or you may end up with a very stiff shoulder and a long series of treatments to loosen it up.

HOME TREATMENT

Treatment involves resting the sore area in combination with exercise to prevent adhesions and stiffness. It's the old problem of rest versus exercise, and you need both in carefully considered amounts.

Rest means take it easy and listen to the pain message. Try not to do things that hurt or that make the pain worse the next day. Avoid the activity that started the whole thing. Common sense will tell you what to do.

Better rest can be obtained with a *sling*. To fashion a sling, you need two big safety pins and a square piece of cloth two to three feet on a side. Fold the cloth diagonally to make a triangle. Put your forearm across the middle of the triangle with your wrist at the right-angle corner. Have a helper tie or pin the free ends of the triangle behind your neck. Pin up the triangular cravat around the elbow as if you were wrapping a package. This simple sling is the most important treatment for everything from a broken shoulder to acute calcific tendinitis. Wear it all the time for the first few days, then decrease use as the pain subsides.

Exercise absolutely must be done, but it must be "passive." You are not trying to build strength but to keep things loose. Work the shoulder through its normal motion in all directions (or as close to that goal as you can come without too much discomfort) several times each day.

Start with "pendulum swings," either dangling your bad arm off the bed or leaning over so that it can hang like a pendulum. Swing it around in little circles and let the circles enlarge. As you get better, you can do this exercise out at the side, where it eventually becomes an "airplane propeller."

Try the gentle hand clap—first in front of your chest, then over your head, then behind your back, then repeat.

To note your progress, do "wall climbing." Here, you stand sideways to a wall about two feet (60 cm) distant and, with arm straight, walk your fingers up the wall. See how high you can get without too much pain. Make a mark, and try to beat it each day.

Aspirin or acetaminophen may be used to decrease pain, but stay free of major pain-killers. If your doctor has prescribed anti-inflammatory drugs, be sure that you are taking them exactly as prescribed.

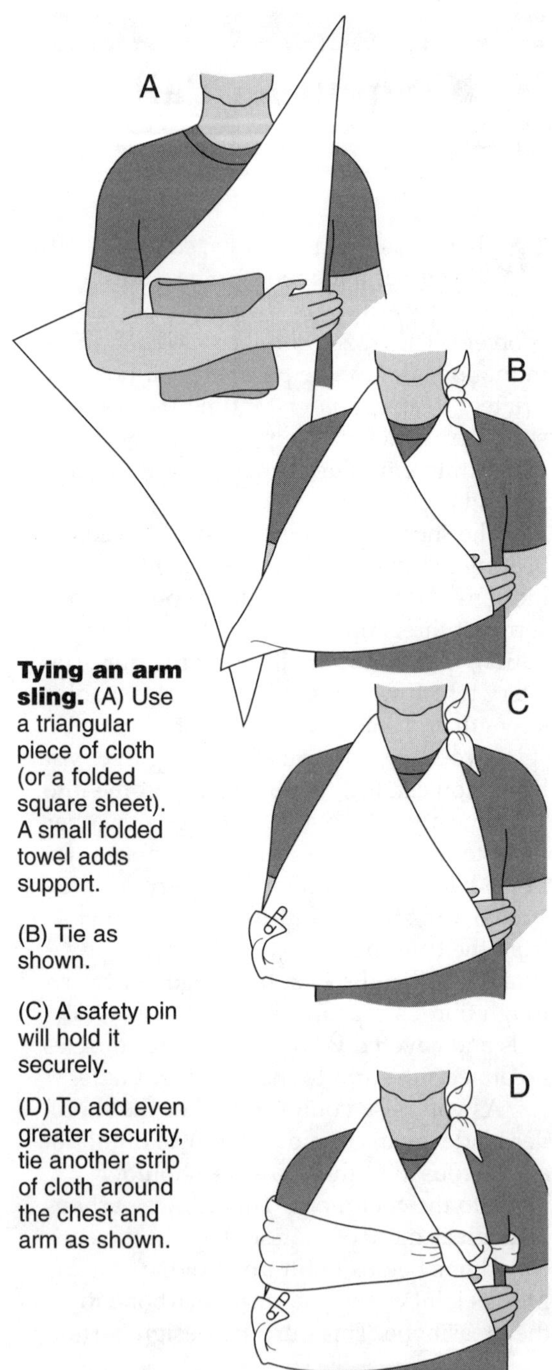

Tying an arm sling. (A) Use a triangular piece of cloth (or a folded square sheet). A small folded towel adds support.

(B) Tie as shown.

(C) A safety pin will hold it securely.

(D) To add even greater security, tie another strip of cloth around the chest and arm as shown.

SHOULDER PAIN

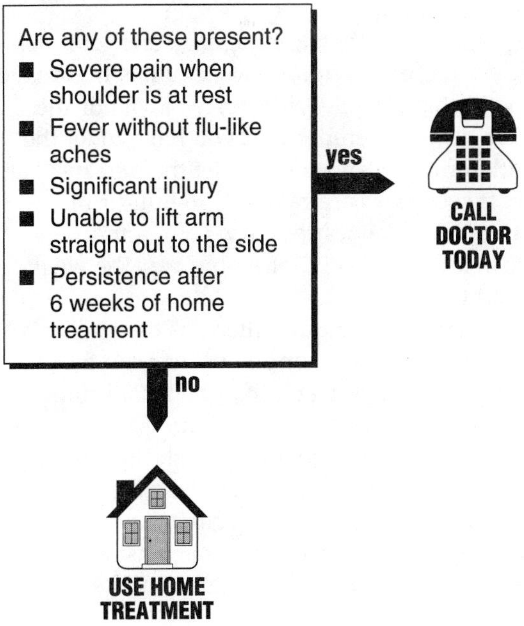

Are any of these present?

- Severe pain when shoulder is at rest
- Fever without flu-like aches
- Significant injury
- Unable to lift arm straight out to the side
- Persistence after 6 weeks of home treatment

yes → **CALL DOCTOR TODAY**

no → **USE HOME TREATMENT**

WHAT TO EXPECT AT THE DOCTOR'S OFFICE

The doctor will examine the shoulder and its range of motion. X-rays may be taken and may show calcium deposits, but this is neither good nor bad and doesn't change the treatment. You may be given an anti-inflammatory drug.

You should be instructed in exercises and you should set up a future appointment to make sure things are going well. If you don't do the exercises or if the doctor isn't familiar with them, you may be sent to a physical therapist for instruction or treatment.

The shoulder may be injected with a steroid—this often helps. In severe cases that have lasted a long time, the joint may be "mobilized under anesthesia" to loosen it up. This rather primitive approach is surprisingly useful. Surgery is not terribly useful in most instances; for example, calcium removal is often unsuccessful. The artificial shoulder joint is a promising approach to severe and persistent problems.

SYMPTOM S15

15 Elbow Pain

The elbow is really two closely related joints. One is a simple hinge joint that operates from straight to about 150 degrees of flexion. The second allows the forearm to twist. The first action allows us to eat, and the second is required to eat soup. Several structures around the elbow may give trouble. Over the point of the elbow is the olecranon bursa, a frequent location for bursitis. On the inside and outside of the elbow are bony bumps to which the muscles attach. These are frequent sites of tendinitis; for example, tennis elbow is a tendinitis on the outside bump. The joint space can be the location of infection or gout; these conditions will cause the part to hurt even though it is not being moved. Young children, usually after being swung by their arms by their parents, sometimes suffer a kind of dislocation. The elbow is exposed enough so that fracture is not uncommon. This injury can be difficult to treat because the bones that usually break are right at the joint.

HOME TREATMENT

Apply rest combined with exercises to prevent stiffness. If you know the cause of the problem, stop doing it. For example, a tennis elbow is caused by a bad, jerky backhand, which puts extra strain where the forearm muscle joins the bone. You can stop tennis for a while, and later you can take some lessons to improve that stroke. For tennis elbow, an elastic strap over the upper forearm (available at tennis shops) will take tension off the sore tendon and can allow healing or even continued play.

Listen for the pain message and let it tell you what not to do. Avoid activities that make the problem worse either right away or the next day. Remember that you have to let the inflammation subside and let the part heal; at least six weeks are required to build full strength. To avoid reinjury, your activity must be below the level that would tear the weakened tendon.

Avoid strong painkillers, as they get in the way of your reception of the pain message. Aspirin or acetaminophen is all right, but they won't help you much.

Rest means take it easy with the elbow. The *sling* (triangular cravat) described in Shoulder Pain **(S14)** is the best way to rest it. Wear the sling every day for at least a few days; it will rest the elbow and will keep you from using it.

Exercise starts from day one. As with the shoulder, we don't want to build strength, we just want to keep the joint loose so that adhesions and stiffness do not result. The most likely deformity is inability to straighten the arm, so we want to pay particular attention to that motion.

Exercise is passive and very simple. Straighten the arm. Let it hang by your side. Flex it and let it straighten out again. Do this at least ten times, twice a day, but don't force too hard at first. Then twist the forearm. Start with your arm extended outward, palm facing the floor, then turn your palm upward to face the ceiling. Repeat ten times, twice a day. If the elbow is really tight, exercise in the shower with warm water running on the elbow. As you get better, do the exercises faster and force them a little harder. But don't force all the way. As soon as you feel the beginning of pain, back off.

ELBOW PAIN

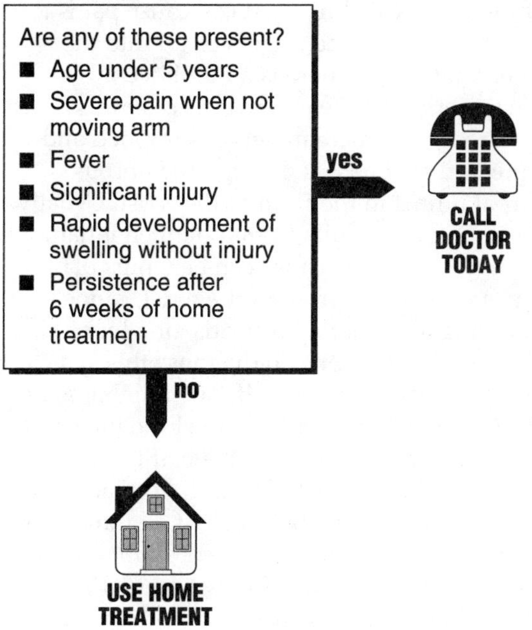

Are any of these present?
- Age under 5 years
- Severe pain when not moving arm
- Fever
- Significant injury
- Rapid development of swelling without injury
- Persistence after 6 weeks of home treatment

yes → **CALL DOCTOR TODAY**

no → **USE HOME TREATMENT**

WHAT TO EXPECT AT THE DOCTOR'S OFFICE

The doctor will examine the elbow and its motion. X-rays are likely if you have had an injury, but they are of little value otherwise. If the elbow is swollen, fluid may be withdrawn through a needle. This is quick, easy, and pretty safe, and can give good information about gout or infection. You may be given a nonsteroidal anti-inflammatory drug, or if you are already taking one, the dosage may be increased. Injection with a corticosteroid can sometimes be helpful if the problem is synovitis in the joint space; it has some hazard if the injection is around a tendon because the tendon can be weakened. At any rate, you shouldn't have more than an occasional injection. Elbows have been destroyed in athletes by repeated injection combined with continuing the activity that caused the problem. Surgery is rarely needed unless there is a fracture, in which case the bones may need to be surgically set and a pin may need to be placed. You may be sent to a physical therapist, but it is usually better for you to do your own exercises regularly than to rely on professional treatment just one or two times a week.

SYMPTOM S16

16 Wrist Pain

The wrist is an unusual joint because stiffness or even fusion causes relatively little difficulty, while lack of stability can pose real problems. The wrist provides the platform from which the fine motions of the fingers operate; it is essential that this platform be stable. The eight wrist bones form a rather crude joint that is very limited in motion compared with, say, the shoulder, but which is strong and stable. Almost no regular human activities require the wrist to be bent all the way back or all the way forward, and the fingers don't operate as well when the wrist is fully flexed or fully extended.

The wrist platform works best when the wrist is bent upward just a little. To illustrate this position, make a fist and put your thumb in the middle of your fist. Holding your arm outstretched at your side and looking down your arm, the thumb should be on an imaginary horizontal line going straight down the middle of your forearm. Thus, any item in your grasp, if the wrist is in proper position, can be pulled or pushed in the most efficient manner.

The wrist can be affected by synovitis, as in rheumatoid arthritis, can be infected, or can be the site of gout or pseudogout. With injury, the wrist may be sprained or the forearm bones may break just above the wrist, the *Colles fracture.* With gonorrhea, the back of the wrist may be inflamed and wiggling the fingers may be painful. This *tenosynovitis* of the wrist may occur together with another clue to VD, a small red skin mark with a little blister in the center.

The *carpal tunnel syndrome* can cause pain at the wrist. In addition, it can cause pains to shoot down into the fingers or up into the forearm. Usually there is a numb feeling in the fingers, as if they were asleep. In this syndrome, the median nerve is trapped and squeezed as it passes through the fibrous carpal tunnel in the front of the wrist. Usually the squeezing results from too much inflammatory tissue. The cause can be tennis playing, a blow to the front of the wrist, canoe paddling, rheumatoid arthritis, or a lot of other problems. You can diagnose this syndrome pretty well yourself. The numbness in the fingers will not involve the little finger and often will not involve the half of the ring finger nearest the little finger. If you tap with a finger on the front of the wrist, you may get a sudden tingling in the fingers similar to the feeling of hitting your "funny bone." Tingling and pain may be worse at night or when the wrists are cocked down.

HOME TREATMENT

A splint is splendid. Since stability is essential and loss of motion is not as serious in the wrist as in other joints, the treatment strategy is a little different. Exercises to increase the motion of the joint are not as important. The strategy is to rest the joint in the position of best function. Wrist splints are available at hospital supply stores and some drugstores. Any that fit you are probably all right. The splint will be of plastic or aluminum, and the hand rest will cock your wrist back just a bit. You can put a cloth sleeve around the splint to make it more comfortable against your skin, and wrap the splint and your arm gently with an elastic bandage to keep it in place. That's all there is to it. Wear it all the time for a few days, then just at night for a few weeks. This simple treatment is all that is required for

WRIST PAIN

Are any of these present?
- Severe pain even when wrist is at rest
- Fever
- Significant injury
- Tingling in the fingers
- Recent exposure to venereal disease (VD)
- Rapid development of swelling without injury
- Persistence after 6 weeks of home treatment

yes

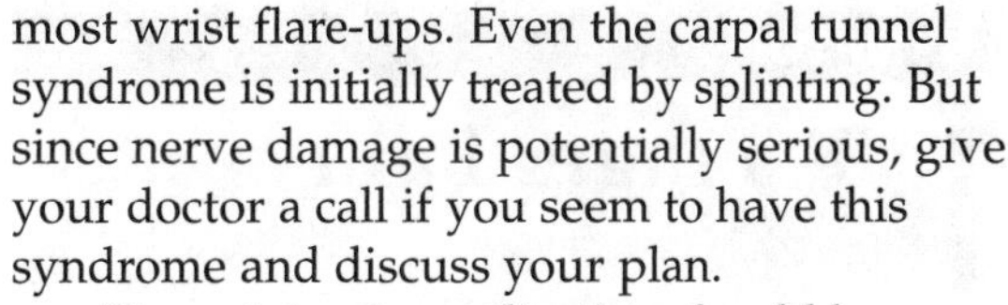

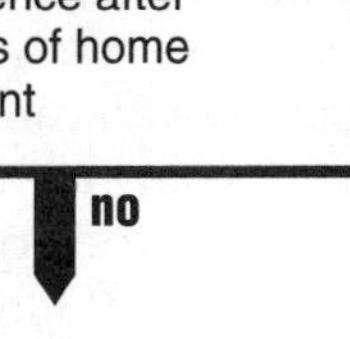

CALL DOCTOR TODAY

no

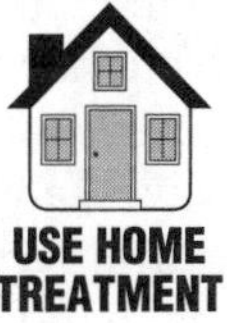

USE HOME TREATMENT

most wrist flare-ups. Even the carpal tunnel syndrome is initially treated by splinting. But since nerve damage is potentially serious, give your doctor a call if you seem to have this syndrome and discuss your plan.

No major pain medication should be necessary; aspirin and similar-strength medications are all right but probably won't help much. If you are taking a prescribed anti-inflammatory drug, be certain that you are taking it just as directed; sometimes a flare-up is due simply to inadequate medication.

If you know what triggered the pain, work out a way to avoid the activity. Common sense means listening to the pain message.

WHAT TO EXPECT AT THE DOCTOR'S OFFICE

Examination of the sore wrist followed by advice similar to that above can be expected. X-rays may be required, but rarely. Anti-inflammatory drugs may be prescribed. Injection with a steroid may be performed on occasion and is likely if a carpal tunnel syndrome has not responded to splinting. Surgery of several different kinds is available, and one or another procedure may be recommended depending on your problem. The carpal tunnel nerve compression may be surgically released. In rheumatoid arthritis, the synovial tissue on the back of the hand may be removed to protect the tendons that run through the inflamed area. The wrist may be casted or fused. Rarely, removal of the ends of the forearm bones will help prevent further damage.

SYMPTOM S17

17 Finger Pain

Each hand has fourteen finger joints, each of which acts like a small hinge. Because the joints are small, they are operated by muscles in the forearm that control the joints by an intricate system of small slings for the tendon leaders. The small size and complicated arrangements mean that any inflammation or damage to the joint is likely to result in some stiffness and lost motion, as even a small adhesion will limit motion.

So you shouldn't expect that a problem with a small finger joint will resolve completely. Even after healing is complete, some leftover stiffness and occasional twinges of discomfort are likely. Unrealistically high expectations lead to feelings that you did something wrong or that the doctor was no good. In fact, almost all of us have a few fingers that have been injured and remain a bit crooked or stiff. The hand functions very well with such deformities; fingers need not open fully or close completely to be perfectly functional.

These small joints are very seldom the location for gout or bacterial infection. But in rheumatoid arthritis, lupus, and other forms of synovitis, the finger joints are often the most affected of any joints. Virus arthritis and drug allergies commonly affect the small finger joints. Osteoarthritis frequently causes knobby swelling of the most distant joints of the fingers. Rheumatoid arthritis usually concentrates on the middle joints and the joints at the near ends of the fingers. Scleroderma can cause loss of motion by tightening of the skin. Sprains, strains, and small fractures are common.

HOME TREATMENT

Listen to the pain message and avoid activities that cause or aggravate pain. Rest the finger joints so that they can heal, but use gentle stretching exercises to keep them limber and maintain motion. You can't cast the fingers very well, and splints tend to leave stiff joints behind, so the key to managing your finger arthritis is to use common sense.

With a bit of ingenuity you can find a less stressful way to do almost any activity that puts stress on the joints. Since everyone's activities are a bit different, you'll have to invent these new ways yourself. Here are a few hints to get you going. A big handle can be gripped with less strain than a small handle, so wrapping pens, knives, and other similar objects with tape or putting a sponge-rubber handle over the original handle can protect your fingers from strain when gripping. Lift smaller loads. Make more trips. Plan ahead rather than blundering through an activity. Let others open the car door for you. Get power steering or a very light car. Use a gripper for opening tough jar lids or stop buying products that come in hard-to-open jars. When opening a tough lid, apply friction pressure on the top of the lid with your palm and twist with your whole hand, not your grip. Cultivate ingenious friends who are handy at making little gadgets to help you. Don't put heavy objects too high or too low. Organize your kitchen, workshop, study, and bedroom to make things easier to grab or move.

Stretch the joints gently twice a day to maintain motion. Straighten the hand out against the tabletop. Make a fist and then cock

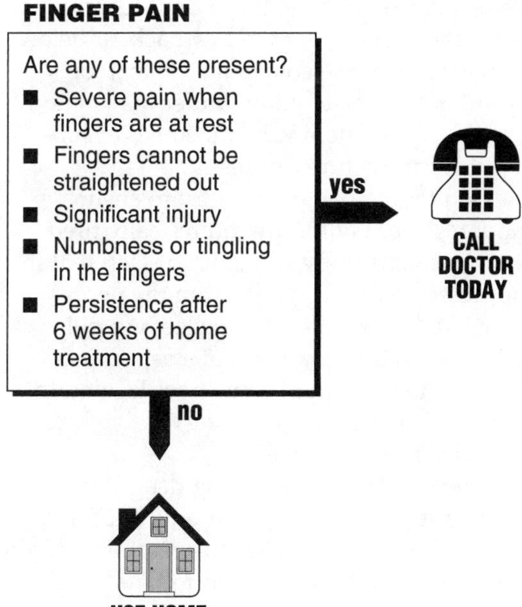

the wrist to increase the stretch. Use one hand to move each finger of the other hand through full flexing to straight out. Don't force, but stretch just to the edge of discomfort. If the motion of a joint is normal, one repetition is enough, but if the motion is limited, do ten repetitions. Warming the hands in warm water before stretching may help you get more motion.

Don't use strong pain medications; they mask the pain so that you may overdo an activity or an exercise. Be sure that you take prescribed medication for inflammation exactly as instructed. Good hand function is important and you want to pay close attention to treatment.

WHAT TO EXPECT AT THE DOCTOR'S OFFICE

The doctor will examine your hands and their motions. Sometimes an X-ray is taken, but usually not more often than every two years. An increase in anti-inflammatory medications may be suggested. Rarely, injection of a particularly bad joint is helpful, but this is less effective with small joints than with large ones. Surgery is also less effective with small joints and isn't indicated often. Surgery, such as placement of plastic joints or removal of inflamed tissue, usually makes the hand look more normal and sometimes decreases the pain, but the hand often doesn't work much better than it did before the operation.

SYMPTOM S18

18 Pain at Night

Night pain is really an indication of the severity of pain. Usually pain will decrease at night as the body diminishes its sensation input for sleep and becomes less active. Typically, a patient with arthritis may have occasional night pains when changing position but will be free of serious discomfort for most of the night. While it may seem that sleep is lost by these brief episodes, the body gets plenty of sleep and no serious problem is present.

Most people overestimate the magnitude of a sleeping problem. Unless the sleeping time totals less than four hours, the body is very good at substituting quality for quantity. The drive to sleep is overwhelming, and the truly tired person will sleep under the most adverse circumstances. Once in a great while, a vicious cycle occurs in which pain prevents sleep, fatigue prevents rational approaches to problems during the day, depression aggravates pain, and sleep is even more disturbed by pain and depression. The hints given here can help with most of these problems.

HOME TREATMENT

Have a comfortable bed. Usually a moderately firm mattress of good quality is the best choice. A waterbed, which supports the weight of the body evenly and can be kept quite warm, is successful for some people with arthritis, while others never can get used to the thing. Pillows can be used here and there to increase comfort. For example, they can be placed on the sides to limit turning, under the neck, under the low back, or below the feet to keep the covers off the feet. Be careful not to use a pillow under the knees if there is any problem with the knees or hips, as a stiff contracture can result.

Don't go to bed early to try to ensure enough sleep. Wait until you're really tired. You want your body so ready to sleep that it suppresses painful signals from the nerves.

Beware of sedatives and sleeping pills. These give the wrong kind of sleep, cause rebound depression in some people, tend to be habit-forming, and only very rarely help solve sleeping problems.

Beware also of painkilling drugs. These do not affect the arthritis but only suppress the symptoms, and the symptom of night pain is one that should be listened to. The body has mechanisms for adjusting to long-term pain, and many doctors feel that pain medications interfere with normal adaptation to pain.

The sleeping partner is important. A restless partner may make twin beds advisable. On the other hand, sexual relations at bedtime encourage good relaxation and healthy sleep.

Be sure to take your anti-inflammatory drugs as prescribed. If your doctor has encouraged you to adjust your own doses, try to be sure that you have a dose at bedtime. Setting the alarm so as to take another dose in the middle of the night may be worthwhile.

PAIN AT NIGHT

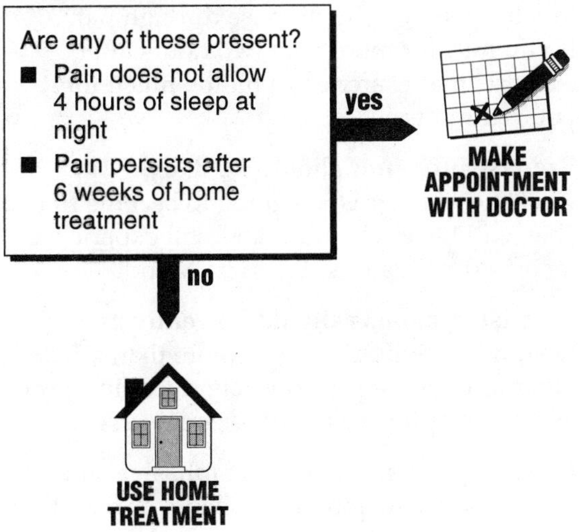

Are any of these present?

- Pain does not allow 4 hours of sleep at night
- Pain persists after 6 weeks of home treatment

yes → **MAKE APPOINTMENT WITH DOCTOR**

no → **USE HOME TREATMENT**

WHAT TO EXPECT AT THE DOCTOR'S OFFICE

The complaint of night pain is a signal to your doctor that your arthritis needs some attention. Examination, tests, even X-rays may be required. A new treatment program may be developed, emphasizing more powerful anti-inflammatory medicines. Most experienced doctors will be cautious with pain medication and sedatives and will try to deal with the underlying problem.

SYMPTOM S19

19 Pain After Exercise

Quite simply, if you are getting pain after exercise, your body is telling you not to do the activity that caused the pain. The pain message is your most important ally as you fight your arthritis. Listen to it.

But there is a paradox: To get better, you have to increase your exercise, and this inevitably will trigger at least a few episodes of increased pain. This pain is not a message to eliminate the exercise program! Rather, it is a suggestion from your body to proceed more carefully with your planned exercise progression. So don't be discouraged by pain after exercise. Listen to it and work with it.

Discomfort immediately after exercise is common with mechanical problems such as strains, fractures, or degenerated cartilage. Inflammatory conditions such as synovitis or attachment arthritis often get better with movement, while mechanical problems get worse. The day after the exercise, almost any form of arthritis or rheumatism may feel worse.

You don't need the doctor unless signs of severe injury or nerve damage are present or unless the problem continues to bother you quite a bit for quite a while. This problem is a signal to review your home exercise program.

HOME TREATMENT

Almost always, pain indicates that you have disregarded one of the principles of a sound exercise program. Let's review them.

Exercise should not make you hurt very much. Don't try to exercise through pain. If you hurt for more than two hours after exercise, that exercise is a bit too much for you right now.

Exercise programs should be daily. The weekend warrior is not going to become fit or able, will have reinjuries, and will experience increased pain and stiffness on Mondays.

Exercise programs should be gently graded. No day's activity should be more than a 10% increase over the previous day's activity. Slow and steady progression is essential to success.

Exercise programs should emphasize smooth actions. Try swimming, walking, or bicycling until good conditioning is achieved. Jerky exercises with incompletely trained muscles are likely to result in reinjury.

Exercise programs for arthritis should emphasize suppleness and muscle tone, not absolute strength. The stress of lifting heavy objects, squeezing balls, and so forth is likely to damage an already injured joint. Swimming easily is the perfect exercise.

Exercise should be preceded by a warm-up period. During warm-up, the joints, ligaments, and muscles are stretched gently. The parts to be used should be physically warm; on a cold day, wear warm-up clothing.

Exercise programs are in addition to, not instead of, prescribed medications. Adherence to prescribed medication programs, particularly with anti-inflammatory drugs, may be essential to your success with exercise.

Now, review your exercise plan, revise it if necessary, and get on with it.

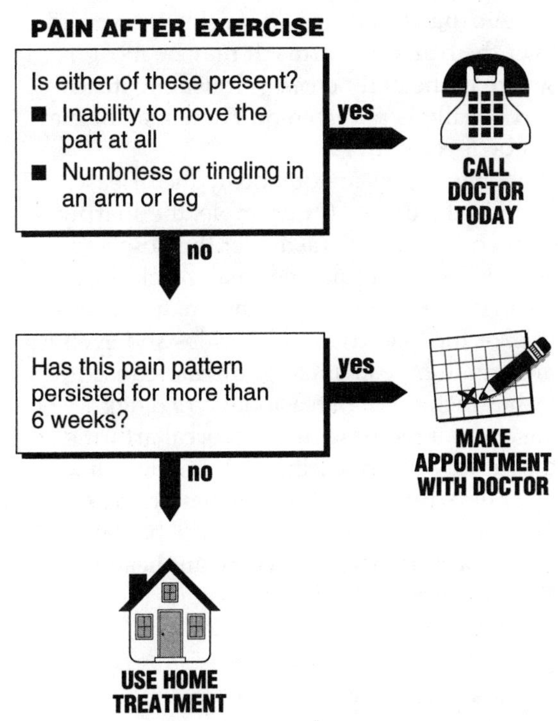

WHAT TO EXPECT AT THE DOCTOR'S OFFICE

The physician will reinforce the concepts reviewed above. If you have trouble figuring out how to apply the principles, you may be referred to a physical therapist. Anti-inflammatory medication might be increased, but this is not necessarily a good idea. Your understanding of the exercise program and of the patience required to recondition your body are essential. Older people are likely to think that serious exercise programs are for the young. This is absolutely not so. The principles of conditioning apply to all ages. You won't get as well as you might unless you persevere in your exercise program.

SYMPTOM **S20**

20 Skin Rash

Allergy is a strong signal to stop the offending medicine. Skin rash and asthmatic attacks are the most common drug allergies, and only skin rash is common with drugs used for arthritis. Still, if you think that wheezing or difficulty in breathing might be due to a drug, then you should call your doctor without delay.

Any new skin rash while on any medication should raise suspicion in your mind. Any drug can cause a rash, and even the "inert" ingredients in tablets have been found to cause rashes. A drug rash can become severe if the drug is continued after the rash has been noticed. So call the doctor before taking any more tablets.

Some drugs are more likely than others to cause rash. In arthritis patients, penicillin or ampicillin are the most frequent rash producers. Although they are not used for treating arthritis very often, they are frequently given to arthritis patients for other reasons. Other antibiotics, including sulfa, are often implicated. Drug-induced lupus may be caused by procaine amide, isoniazid (INH), hydralazine, and other drugs. Allopurinol causes skin rash in up to 3% of persons taking this drug. Toxic reactions to oral or intramuscular gold and penicillamine may involve skin rash, often with mouth ulcers as well.

On the other hand, some drugs are pretty unlikely to cause rash. Aspirin, acetaminophen (Tylenol), hydroxychloroquine (Plaquenil), colchicine, and prednisone hardly ever cause a rash.

A drug rash is usually fairly widespread over the trunk and arms. It may be most severe in the body creases. It usually itches and usually is red in color. There may or may not be fever with it.

Some rashes are obviously the disease and not the drug—for example, the sharply defined "butterfly" rash over the nose and cheeks seen in lupus, the small black sores at the corners of the nails in rheumatoid arthritis, or the lilac-colored knuckles and eyelids in dermatomyositis. Other disease-caused rashes include the occasional "fried egg" blister on a red base in gonococcal arthritis, the rapidly disappearing rash on the trunk in juvenile arthritis, scaling patches on the soles in Reiter's syndrome, and painful blisters in one part of the body with complicating "shingles." Pitted nails and scaling patches are characteristic of psoriatic arthritis.

HOME TREATMENT

The easiest rash of all to cure is a drug rash. Usually it will be very much better within two days; all you do is stop the drug after talking with your doctor, and wait. If the rash itches a lot, a warm bath with two tablespoons (30 cc) of baking soda in it can help. If the rash persists, check again with your doctor. Tell your doctor about any possible drug rash; you may need new medication or perhaps some tests for allergic damage to other organs.

WHAT TO EXPECT AT THE DOCTOR'S OFFICE

The drug will be stopped if there is a reasonable suspicion that it is causing the rash. If possible, the doctor will keep you off all drugs for a while; often a suspected allergic reaction is a good chance to review the entire treatment program. New drugs, with different

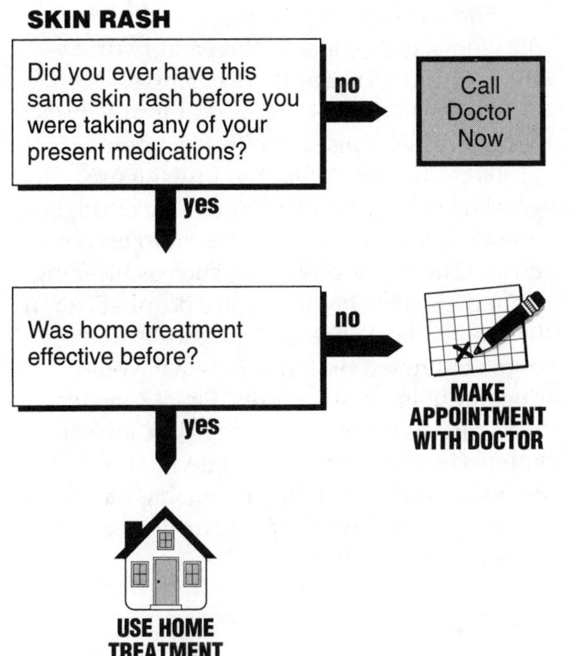

chemical formulas so that they will not "cross-react," may be prescribed. Drugs may be reintroduced carefully, one at a time, if several are suspected. Blood tests for liver or kidney damage may be suggested.

SYMPTOM S21

21 Nausea or Vomiting

Nausea and vomiting have a whole host of causes. Of course there is the flu. Or it may be ulcers, food poisoning, gallbladder problems, or motion sickness. On the other hand, if you're taking a drug for arthritis and have nausea or vomiting, chances are that the drug is responsible.

Most stomach problems from drugs are due to direct irritation of the stomach lining. If you look in the stomach with a gastroscope, you may see an area of gastritis with the pill sitting in the middle of the inflamed area. Some of the drugs that can cause gastritis also can cause nausea by certain effects on the brain, but the direct irritation is almost always the major problem. Direct irritant drugs include aspirin, Indocin, Motrin, Nalfon, Naprosyn, Tolectin, Feldene, and Clinoril, among others.

Some other drugs wreak havoc on your gastrointestinal tract differently. Prednisone and other steroids seem to increase the acid in the stomach while decreasing the mucus layer that protects the stomach lining. Colchicine usually causes diarrhea, but a few patients experience nausea as well. Gold salts and penicillamine sometimes cause ulcers in the mouth or stomach wall that are not due to direct toxicity but can result in nausea or vomiting.

Finally, some powerful immunosuppressant drugs seem to cause nausea by interfering with cell division and cell repair in the stomach and small intestine. These drugs include Imuran, methotrexate, and chlorambucil.

Some drugs are generally pretty safe for the stomach. Acetaminophen and hydroxychloroquine (Plaquenil) are examples.

Home treatment works best for the direct irritant drugs. This side effect is a double problem; you don't want to lose the use of a good drug because of a minor side effect, but you also don't want the problem to become major. The major problems, such as bleeding from the stomach, can require hospitalization or even be fatal. The best practice is to try home treatment first. If it fails, ask your doctor for some more hints. Finally, switch medications if your stomach is just too sensitive. Good judgment is needed to know when to stop a drug that is causing nausea or stomach pain. Check with your doctor if you aren't sure what to do.

HOME TREATMENT

If your doctor has told you to take the suspected drug only if you need it, try stopping the drug for a few days and start over with a more comfortable stomach. If your doctor wants you to take the medicine regularly, then try these tricks. Space the same dose out through the day. For example, instead of two tablets every four hours, try one tablet every two hours. Take at least an eight-ounce (250 ml) glass of water with each dose to dilute the chemical in the stomach. Take the drug after meals, when the food in the stomach will help protect the stomach lining. Or take one ounce (30 ml) of a liquid antacid (such as Maalox, Gelusil, or Riopan) a few minutes before you take the medication dose. Tums or OsCal, up to four a day, may also work, and will also help your calcium intake.

If these don't work, try around-the-clock buffering. Eat six small meals a day instead of three big ones. Keep something in the stomach each hour when awake; if this is not a

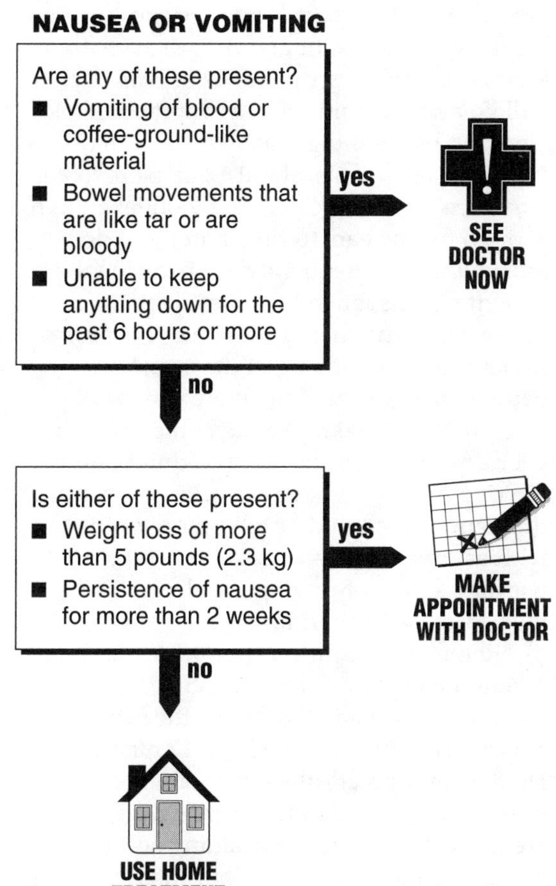

meal, then make it an ounce (30 ml) of antacid. Set the alarm to go off during the night, take some antacid, and then reset the alarm for a few hours later. Check with the doctor if you don't seem to be making good progress; this regimen should make you more comfortable in just a couple of days.

Remember that side effects are to be expected from drugs. We just have to keep them at the level of minor annoyances, not major problems.

WHAT TO EXPECT AT THE DOCTOR'S OFFICE

The doctor will ask some questions and may have some further suggestions. If the problem is major you may have to have a gastroscopy (interior examination of the stomach) or an X-ray of the stomach. Usually, however, it is simpler just to stop the drug. Your doctor will try to suggest a medication that will cause less irritation and do the same job for your arthritis.

SYMPTOM S22

22 Ringing in the Ears

Aspirin is the most likely cause of this problem. The second most likely cause is aspirin. So is the third. Possibly, other anti-inflammatory drugs cause *tinnitus,* which is the medical word for "ringing in the ears," but aspirin is overwhelmingly the major cause.

This is a warning sign of aspirin toxicity. It means that the aspirin level in your blood is approaching the upper margin of safety. If you take more aspirin, the sequence of events is something like this. The first ringing is mild and is noticed about one to two hours after the last dose. Then the ringing becomes louder and constant. Hearing begins to decrease, and the ringing may seem to improve simply because you can't hear it as well. You experience shortness of breath and begin to breathe hard and fast. You now have moderately severe aspirin toxicity.

Serious aspirin toxicity is rare in adults. It is more frequently seen in children who manage to get into the "childproof" bottles. Don't be frightened by the sequence above; aspirin remains one of our safer medications. All drugs are subject to overuse, and aspirin is no exception.

When you stop the aspirin, the aspirin level in your blood begins to decrease and will decline slowly over several days. As it goes down, the sequence will reverse. Damage is not permanent, except for very rare hearing damage in very severe cases. If you had a damaged liver before the episode, the aspirin may remain in your blood even longer, since the liver acts to remove the aspirin from the body. If you are short of breath, call the doctor and discuss the situation. It is probably due to the aspirin and will go away within the day, but it could always be something else.

For most people, about 12 or more tablets a day are required to get the blood level high enough for the ears to ring, and these doses are now used infrequently. An occasional patient reports it at a lower level, but such instances often reflect patient nervousness rather than true ringing of the ears. Some people don't get ringing before 40 tablets (200 grains, 13,000 mg) a day; other people get decreased hearing first and don't notice the ringing. If you have a preexisting hearing problem, you should be a bit more careful with aspirin, since you might not get the warning signal of ringing. Be alert for a further decrease in hearing.

Remember, aspirin is in a wide variety of patent medicines. The terms ASA, aspirin, and acetylsalicylic acid all describe the same drug. Anacin, Bufferin, Alka-Seltzer, Contac, APCs, Dristan, and practically every other cold tablet or pain reliever contains aspirin. Exceptions are those medications containing acetaminophen, such as Tylenol, or ibuprofen, such as Advil or Nuprin.

HOME TREATMENT

Stop all aspirin-containing medication and wait for the ringing to go away. This may take only two hours or it may take two days. Ringing in the ears is *not* a reason to stop the medication permanently. It is merely a signal to use a somewhat lower dose. So gradually start the medication again and keep to a slightly lower dose. If your ears rang the first time at 16 tablets a day, try 14. If they ring again at 14, try 12. Ringing will be less and arthritis will benefit more if you spread the

RINGING IN THE EARS

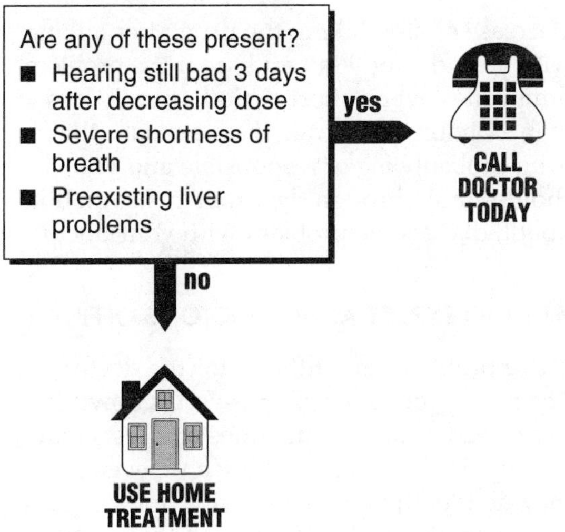

Are any of these present?
- Hearing still bad 3 days after decreasing dose
- Severe shortness of breath
- Preexisting liver problems

yes → **CALL DOCTOR TODAY**

no → **USE HOME TREATMENT**

doses out over the whole day as best you can, rather than taking a few large doses of four or five tablets at once.

Ringing in the ears is a good sign. It means that your body absorbs the aspirin well and that you can get good blood levels in order to decrease the inflammation. You are likely to get a good result from your aspirin treatment after the dose is adjusted appropriately.

WHAT TO EXPECT AT THE DOCTOR'S OFFICE

The preceding advice will be repeated by your physician. If your problem is severe, blood tests of liver and kidney function may be done. Doctors are encouraged by this complaint because it indicates a patient who can be counted on to take a prescribed medication. Ringing in the ears happens to the "best" patients.

SYMPTOM S23

23 Dizziness or Headache

These problems have a lot of different possible causes, and you may want to check out the more general discussion that appears in *Take Care of Yourself.* Here we want to make the point that these problems can be the side effects of drugs given for arthritis. You should always be ready to suspect any drug of anything, but there are certain circumstances in which dizziness or headache are most likely to be drug related.

Aspirin in high doses of 12 or more tablets (3,900 mg) daily can cause dizziness and light-headedness in addition to ringing in the ears **(S22).**

Indomethacin (Indocin) is the most notorious of arthritis drugs with regard to these problems. Severe headaches, dizziness, and feelings of detachment are common, particularly in the first few weeks of taking the medication. Usually, but not always, this problem gets better after you have taken the indomethacin for a while.

Less frequently, other anti-inflammatory drugs can cause these problems.

Painkillers, including codeine, Percodan, Darvon, and Talwin, can cause dizziness and unusual "drugged" mental sensations but do not cause head pain.

HOME TREATMENT

Decrease or stop taking the drug after talking with your doctor. Wait and see if the problem diminishes over a short period, usually less than 24 hours. If the dizziness persists, the drug probably is not responsible and you should think through the problem again. If in doubt, discuss the problem with your doctor.

WHAT TO EXPECT AT THE DOCTOR'S OFFICE

These problems are difficult for the doctor. The most problematical question is how far to proceed with investigations and tests that usually don't reveal anything and, even if they do identify an abnormality, don't suggest a good treatment. Often these problems persist for some time on and off but still don't amount to anything major.

In addition to drug causes, nervousness or anxiety, low blood pressure, vertigo, virus, tension, depression, brain tumor, stroke, ear infection, or a hundred other possible causes may be to blame. Skull X-rays usually do not help in a diagnosis. Brain-wave tests, arteriograms, and blood tests usually aren't much help either. So the decisions are difficult. You often can help by not pushing the doctor to do more and more. Just how much investigation is appropriate depends on how long you have had the problem, how much of a problem it poses in your daily life, and what other problems you are having at the same time.

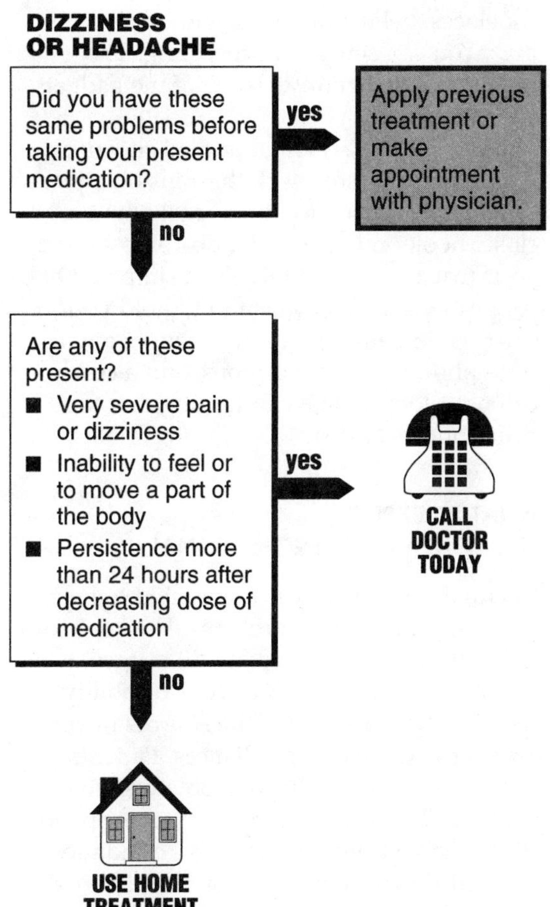
DIZZINESS
OR HEADACHE
Did you have these same problems before taking your present medication?
yes
Apply previous treatment or make appointment with physician.
no
Are any of these present?
■ Very severe pain or dizziness
■ Inability to feel or to move a part of the body
■ Persistence more than 24 hours after decreasing dose of medication
yes
CALL DOCTOR TODAY
no
USE HOME TREATMENT

SYMPTOM S24

24 Difficulty Getting Dressed

Problems with dressing are usually related to the fine finger movements needed to fasten small buttons, the shoulder action necessary to get clothes over the head or to fasten garments behind the back, or the difficulty in reaching the feet to put on trousers, shoes, or socks. Some people may have trouble pulling open a dresser drawer or getting to the dresser.

While patients with rheumatoid arthritis most frequently have problems of this kind, a young man with low back pain or a child with a broken elbow faces the same challenges for a shorter time.

HOME TREATMENT

The idea is to make everything as easy as possible. Put the dresser near the bed. Use a dresser of lightweight wood with small, well-lubricated drawers. Replace small knobs with big handles.

Select clothes that are easy to put on: slip-on shoes, front-fastening garments, zippers with big ring pulls, wraparound robes, clothes with Velcro fasteners, clip-on ties, stretch belts that hook rather than buckle.

Get a helpful friend—or several. A spouse is fine, or a friend with whom you can exchange tasks, each of you doing what you are good at. A friendly handyperson and someone who can use a sewing machine, if you cannot, can be very helpful. Velcro, a marvelous material that sticks to itself simply by applying slight pressure and pulls apart just as easily, can be a wonderful replacement for buttons, shoelaces, belts, bra hooks, and other fastenings. You can sew it on everything. The handyperson can make some of the gadgets you may need.

Get gadgets. A long-handled shoehorn, garter snaps or spring clothespins on a piece of tape for helping to put on socks, and a closet hook on the end of a dowel to extend your reach can make life much simpler. Other suggestions are a valet stand to hold your shirt while you put an arm through, a wire buttonhook for small buttons, and a collar extender loop to make buttoning that top collar button easier.

WHAT TO EXPECT FROM THE HEALTH PROFESSIONAL

Occupational therapists are trained to help you with this kind of problem. The key word is "adaptive"; the therapist will suggest ways in which you can adapt to your disability. The therapist will also know the sources in your area for gadgets and appliances. Patients with a long-term arthritis problem should consider *The Arthritis Helpbook* (see Appendix B), available from the Arthritis Foundation or the Arthritis Society or at your local bookstore. It is a gold mine of hints, pictures, and sources for materials.

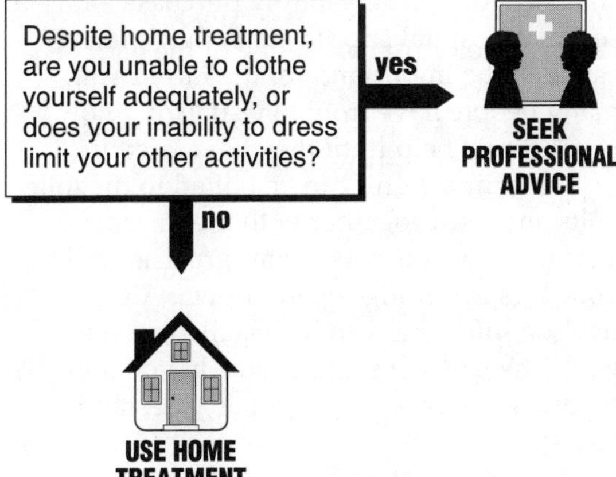
GETTING DRESSED
Despite home treatment, are you unable to clothe yourself adequately, or does your inability to dress limit your other activities?
yes
SEEK PROFESSIONAL ADVICE
no
USE HOME TREATMENT

SYMPTOM S25

25 Problems Using the Toilet

Dignity is a crucial part of the problem here since we usually don't feel comfortable asking another person to help us with our eliminations. So this problem very often goes unmentioned. However, with a few fairly simple measures, a lot of difficulty can be avoided.

Remember, the idea is to make necessary daily activities as easy as possible. This is a sensible idea for everybody, of course, but if you have a physical limitation, the defects in the way our society is designed suddenly become very obvious. What is merely an annoyance for others is a real nuisance to you. And if you can save a few seconds (and some energy) at tasks you must repeat many times, the saving becomes substantial.

The biggest problem is usually the effort involved in getting on and off of the toilet. Muscle weakness in the legs, contractures of the hips, and arthritis of the knees all act to make getting up and down a problem. We discouraged deep knee bends earlier because they stress the knees too much; the action involved in using the toilet is almost the same.

Persons with arthritis of the wrist sometimes have trouble using toilet paper. And a problem with the bowels, whether it is diarrhea or constipation, can make the whole thing more difficult than it need be.

HOME TREATMENT

You need some physical aids. The most important one is a raised toilet seat. In a major remodeling, you can install toilets that are three to five inches (8 to 13 cm) higher than standard, or you can simply purchase a raised seat at a hospital supply store. Don't underestimate the importance of the raised seat; many people have trouble visualizing how much it will help until they have tried it.

An armrest unit can be bolted to the toilet bolts and used together with the raised seat. This permits you to use your arms as well as your legs in getting up and down. Alternatively, a safety bar can be installed on the wall. The bar will serve to steady you and to take some of your weight as you stand and sit.

Severely affected persons can use a glider commode to put a toilet in a nearby location, but we don't find too much use for these. Sometimes they encourage a person to be bedbound when he or she could be more active.

For holding toilet paper, your reach can be extended by a variety of different gadgets. You can make tissue holders from spring-loaded clothespins or coat hangers, or use tongs with plastic tips.

Finally, if money is no object, a bidet can be installed. There are portable bidets that attach to an existing toilet, or entire new units can be installed. These use a jet of warm water to cleanse gently. Although relatively rare in the United States, bidets are commonplace in Europe.

Diarrhea or constipation contribute to the problem of using the toilet, either because of increased frequency or increased straining. So healthy habits (but not obsessions with bowel frequency) are important. A good diet that includes plenty of fruits and vegetables as well as bran and whole wheat breads should be a habit. Exercise regularly and avoid laxatives. If a medication must be taken, use Metamucil—a teaspoonful (5 cc) in a glass of water twice a day. This will increase bulk and stabilize the stool.

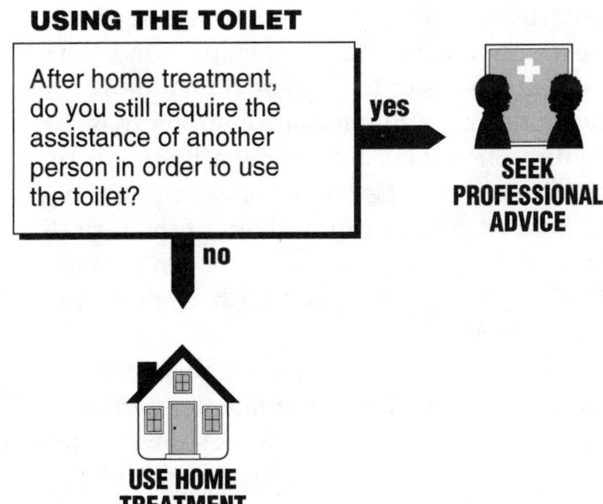

WHAT TO EXPECT FROM THE HEALTH PROFESSIONAL

The occupational therapist may well have some additional hints for you and will know the sources for any purchases you may need. The therapist might visit your home; if so, take advantage of this visit to inquire about hints for the other rooms of your house or apartment.

The social worker may be able to find a source of funds to pay for those things that are too costly for you. Remember that any expenditures you must make to equip your house because of your arthritis are tax deductible; ask your doctor for a prescription for the raised toilet seat, safety bar, or other aid on your next visit. The tax people might want to see it. Your doctor will appreciate your not making a special trip just to obtain such documentation.

Bathroom convenience. A raised toilet seat or commode over the toilet provides greater height and thus makes standing up easier.

SYMPTOM S26

26 Problems with Bathing and Hygiene

These activities are closely tied in to how we feel about ourselves, giving them an importance beyond the medical requirement for decent hygiene. We feel helpless and humiliated if we cannot keep ourselves looking clean or if we must worry about the way we may smell, and these worries may cause us to withdraw from social activities. So these are crucial concerns. The success of other activities may depend on how well we can adapt to problems with bathing, hygiene, and grooming. Some major changes in the home may be necessary for patients with severe arthritis, but the rewards can be dramatic.

Problems usually center on how to get in or out of a tub or shower, or how to hold a toothbrush or comb, or how to reach all parts of the body. The modern house is not very well designed for efficient living, and the patient with arthritis needs to live as efficiently as possible. So you may have to be quite resourceful and do some inventing.

HOME TREATMENT

For a bathtub, mount rails on the wall to help you get in and out safely. Safety rails that mount on the side of the tub are available at hospital supply stores. A suction-cup mat or nonskid tape on the bottom of the tub can prevent you from slipping.

A shower is better for many people, but again use the nonskid tape for safety. An adjustable shower head that moves up and down on a metal rod often helps. Single-lever faucets are easier to manage than old-fashioned ones that require a strong twist to turn on and keep dripping after you turn them off. Don't use soap dishes or plumbing to hold onto; they can pull out of the wall. A sitting shower is possible if you can't stand for long; use a bath bench with suction cups on the legs.

Put the soap in a cloth bag on a string around your neck to eliminate that terrible search for the dropped soap. A shower caddy hanging from the shower head is useful to keep shampoo and brushes close by. A back scrubbing strap can make that chore easy—and it feels good. A bath mitt can help in scrubbing. To dry off, just put on a terry-cloth robe and let it soak up the water.

Put built-up handles on combs, toothbrushes, and hairbrushes. It is much easier to grasp a large handle than a small one. An electric toothbrush can save some effort. If reach is a problem, mount long handles on combs and brushes. You can build up nail clippers with longer wooden handles to make them easier to use. If you mount a nailbrush on suction cups, it will stay put while you scrub.

A "bed bath," requiring only a washcloth, a container of soapy water, a container of clean water, and a towel can satisfactorily reduce the frequency with which you need the full bath or shower.

An electric razor is often more manageable than a hand one, and razor holders to improve your grip are available from major manufacturers such as Remington, Sunbeam, and Norelco.

Many women prefer a cream-type depilatory for their legs. Sanitary napkins are available with adhesive strips that are easy to fasten. There are even Velcro hair curlers that

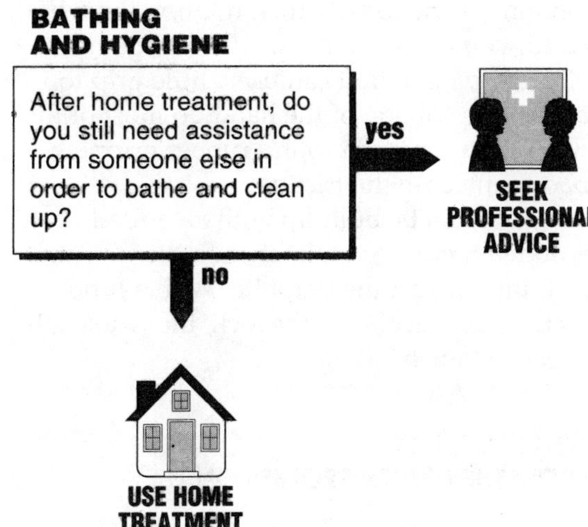

can be worked with one hand. You won't need to make use of all of these tricks, of course, but they are included to give you an idea of the many ways in which you can simplify an essential everyday activity.

WHAT TO EXPECT FROM THE HEALTH PROFESSIONAL

The occupational therapist can suggest additional ideas and will know where to obtain needed gadgets. The social worker can sometimes help in obtaining funds or in finding used equipment. Remember that devices required for your arthritis can be tax deductible, which decreases the cost to you. These expenditures are worth the cost.

The Arthritis Helpbook (see Appendix B) has lots of additional suggestions.

SYMPTOM S27

27 Turning Handles and Opening Doors

When you have arthritis, the world can sometimes seem like an unfriendly place. Design for style rather than for function makes many things difficult even if you have a good thumb and a strong grip. And if you don't, you're in trouble.

Some of these design features are really totally unnecessary. Before you buy, check for good functional design. The key words are *safe, sturdy, efficient, easy to work, easy to fix.* Look for these features when you buy a house, a motor home, a car, shoes, a toothbrush, or anything else. As a consumer, you speak with your dollars—and that's the language the designers ultimately listen to. When you run into something particularly outrageous, write the manufacturer. Write a consumer group. Write a government consumer agency. Keep the pressure on.

Meanwhile, here are a few hints to help you with the world as it is now.

HOME TREATMENT

A handle with pointed bars, like some shower handles, can be worked with a lever—a bamboo or aluminum tube works well. When you buy new fixtures, however, get ones with a single lever that controls both water force and temperature. Remember the lever, because it is the answer to a lot of frustrating problems.

When you grip, learn to use the palm. If you press on a handle, you get a surprising amount of friction. By then rotating the whole hand, you can turn the handle without actually gripping it. You can use a little grip too, but let the friction of the hand do most of the work. You can get a round rubber gripping pad to increase the friction.

Keys can be built up with an added wooden handle to make them easier to turn. But don't forget the graphite. With a little lock oil or graphite in the lock, the whole job becomes much easier.

WHAT TO EXPECT FROM THE HEALTH PROFESSIONAL

The occupational therapist can give you additional adaptive suggestions and is a good person to ask about where to obtain some of the materials you need. *The Arthritis Helpbook* (see Appendix B) is a useful aid to locating ideas and resources.

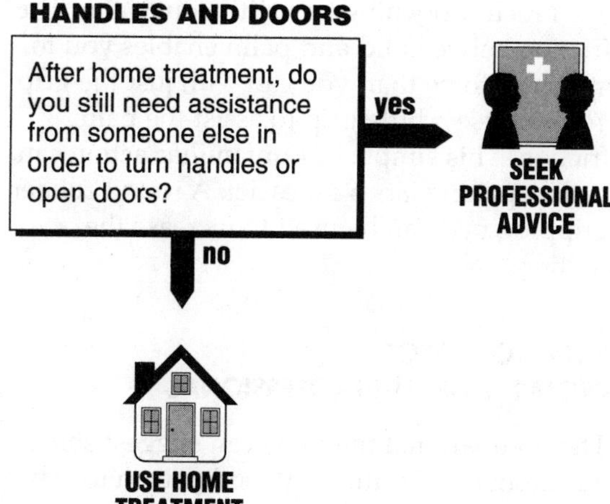
HANDLES AND DOORS
After home treatment, do you still need assistance from someone else in order to turn handles or open doors?
yes
SEEK PROFESSIONAL ADVICE
no
USE HOME TREATMENT

SYMPTOM **S28**

28 Problems Opening Jars

Some people think that applesauce jars are the worst. Others give the award to catsup bottles. Then there are the can openers, and the plastic or cellophane that won't tear. These are problems for everyone. Domestic battles rage over the opening of a difficult jar on a difficult day. And if your grip strength is decreased because of arthritis, you may need some tricks to help you out (with the jars, not the domestic battles).

Don't minimize this problem because it seems so ordinary and so unimportant. Frustration at a trivial task is more marked than with a larger one. Your feeling of helplessness before a stubborn jar is not good for you. So learn the tricks.

HOME TREATMENT

Mount a wedge-shaped gripper on the kitchen wall; this allows you to turn the jar easily with two hands while the lid is securely held. Break the suction on vacuum lids, such as applesauce, with a "lid lifter" available in housewares departments everywhere. Use a fork handle as a lever to pull up ring-top openers.

With boxes, lay the box on its side and cut the top off with a knife. Use scissors for sealed plastic or cellophane.

Get an electric can opener. The ones that have a power stroke to pierce the can will save you additional effort. If you use a hand can opener, make sure the handle is large and easy to grip.

Practice opening jars with your palm. The friction between lid and palm enables you to get more force than you can with just the grip. You can use a little grip to assist the palm friction. This simple but unfamiliar action can make opening jars a lot easier. A round rubber gripping pad can be used to increase the friction.

WHAT TO EXPECT FROM THE HEALTH PROFESSIONAL

The occupational therapist can suggest some additional tricks and is a good person to ask for places to obtain items. Everything you need to conquer this particular problem is probably available at a nearby store, so the health professional will not be of as much assistance. You have to learn to look for items with care, anticipating how well they will work with your particular disability.

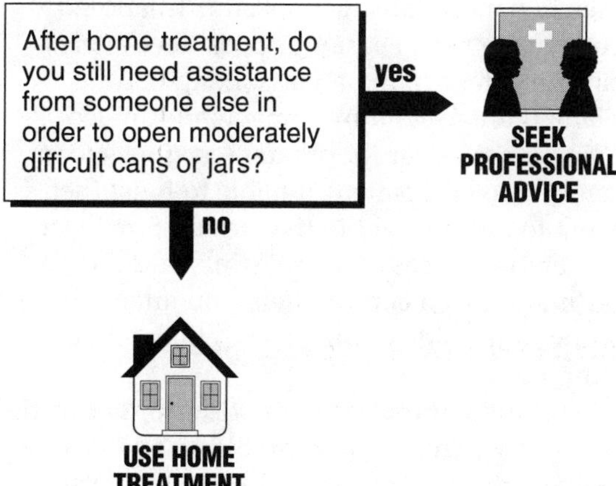
OPENING JARS
After home treatment, do you still need assistance from someone else in order to open moderately difficult cans or jars?
yes
SEEK PROFESSIONAL ADVICE
no
USE HOME TREATMENT

SYMPTOM S29

29 Difficulty with Eating

This is a most fundamental frustration. Eating is a complicated task that involves mental activity, physical abilities, and body reflexes to carry the food to and through the stomach. Interruption of the sequence at any point can cause a problem. The problem for the person with arthritis may involve difficulty in cutting the food, in getting the food to the mouth, in chewing, or in swallowing. These problems affect only a very few patients with arthritis, but they are serious ones. Eating is a social occasion as well as a biological necessity, and eating gracefully without self-consciousness is a social skill we take for granted.

HOME TREATMENT

The suggestions here are just to get you started. As with other daily activities, your own solutions will require a bit of personal input and ingenuity.

There are several ways to make it easier to cut your food. Attractive utensils are available with big handles that enable you to get a better grip. If the plate is placed on a damp sponge cloth, high-friction plastic, or a thin disk of rubber, it will not slip while you are cutting. These measures can help in stirring or opening as well as in cutting, and can give a feeling of greater security. Don't forget that a sharp knife will cut more easily than a dull one. Or that foods can be selected that are equally good in taste but easier to cut.

In getting the food to the mouth, built-up utensil handles are again useful. T-handled cups make for an easier grip, as does a terry-cloth coaster around a glass. Long-handled utensils are needed by some, while angled utensils are easier for others. A swivel spoon can be used by patients unable to twist their wrist to bring liquid to the mouth. Straws are sometimes an easy way to drink, and an ordinary pencil clip can help you attach the straw to the side of the glass to make it even simpler.

Chewing problems can arise from arthritis of the jaw joints or from problems with the teeth or the chewing muscles. Good dental care is essential. Selection of food that can be easily chewed is one way to avoid the problem.

Swallowing can be affected in several ways. In myositis the upper swallowing muscles may not work. In scleroderma the muscles in the lower gullet may not pass a smooth swallowing wave. Medicines given for arthritis may irritate the stomach and not let food leave the stomach efficiently. Chew carefully and slowly, and swallow carefully. If the problem seems to be low in the gullet, an antacid may be helpful. Take small, frequent meals, use softer textured foods, take liquids with meals, and eat and chew slowly. Try not eating for the two or three hours before bedtime if you have pain behind the breastbone when you eat. Having pain when you eat is an indication that you should see the doctor, as is any weight loss due to difficulty eating.

DIFFICULTY WITH EATING

Are any of these present?

- Weight loss over 5 pounds (2.3 kg)
- Significant pain when eating
- After home treatment you still need someone to assist you in order to eat

yes → **SEEK PROFESSIONAL ADVICE**

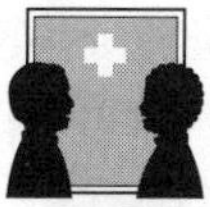

no → **USE HOME TREATMENT**

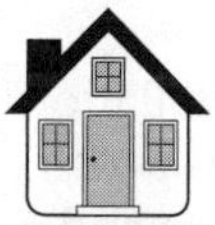

WHAT TO EXPECT FROM THE HEALTH PROFESSIONAL

The occupational therapist is knowledgeable about adaptive aids and where to get them. The social worker may be needed in severe cases to locate public resources. The doctor is necessary if chewing or swallowing problems are causing major difficulty. X-rays of the jaw and the temporomandibular joint may be taken. An upper-GI series is an X-ray of the esophagus, stomach, and duodenum, and it may help identify a problem in these areas.

SYMPTOM S30

30 Problems with Stairs

In some living environments, there is no need to use stairs. This is true of the single-level house or homes equipped with elevators. In other situations, the ability to climb stairs is essential to independent life. Stairs sometimes must be used several times a day; even the bathroom, if upstairs, can require this activity.

Problems with the knees, the hips, or the quadriceps muscles in the thigh are usually responsible for difficulty with stairs. Thus, loss of the ability to climb stairs is a signal for increased attention to your arthritis; a minor problem has just become major.

HOME TREATMENT

Often your first approach should be to check the treatment program for your arthritis. Are you taking the medication regularly? Does your doctor have further suggestions? Are you working on your quadriceps-strengthening exercises? Might a steroid injection of an inflamed knee be of benefit? Is this the signal to consider seriously a surgical procedure on the bad hip or knee?

Sometimes you can rearrange your environment quite a bit. Should you move? An apartment with an elevator? A ranch-style house? Should you remodel? A downstairs bedroom and bath? A ramp in the garden, gently graded? Such changes can sometimes render the stairs unnecessary.

Can you improve the stairs? Be sure you have a rail or banister on each side, so that you can both steady yourself and push a bit with your arms. Sometimes installation of a center rail will help you by allowing you to use both hands at once. The split riser trick also helps some people. If your problem is that the steps are just too high, you can have a carpenter install split risers, so that half of each step is raised half a step, alternating left and right. Then you can climb the stairs, moving back and forth, without ever having to go up a full step at a time.

The rule for climbing stairs: one at a time, with both feet on the same stair before trying the next one. Go up with the good leg first; go down with the good leg first. Use the same technique for curbs.

Another possibility is installation of a home elevator or lift that goes up on a banister. These are fairly expensive and are thus out of reach for all but a few. If you are considering one of these, you should reconsider the option of moving or remodeling.

WHAT TO EXPECT FROM THE HEALTH PROFESSIONAL

The occupational therapist may have some additional suggestions for you and will know where to obtain materials and help. The social worker may be able to help with sources of financing. Remember that changes in your living arrangements, like stairs, necessitated by your arthritis are tax deductible. Thus, the actual cost will be a little less than you first expect.

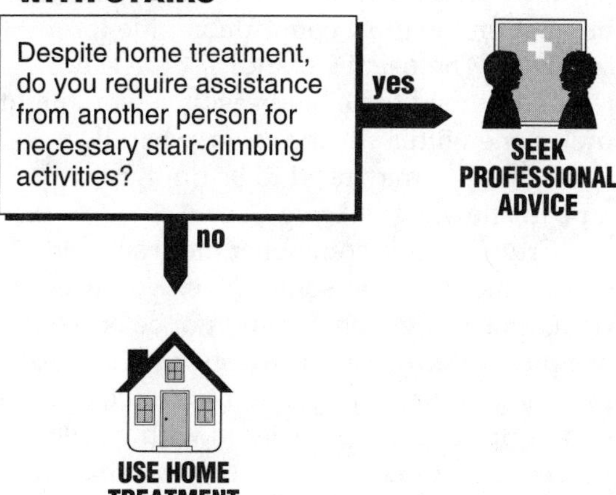
PROBLEMS
WITH STAIRS
Despite home treatment, do you require assistance from another person for necessary stair-climbing activities?
yes
SEEK
PROFESSIONAL
ADVICE
no
USE HOME
TREATMENT

SYMPTOM S31

31 Difficulty Walking

Walking is central to almost every other activity. The ability to walk must be preserved. If walking is impaired, the muscles become weak, the bones lose calcium, friends are more distant, and the easiest tasks become formidable. This cycle can further reduce your health and increase your dependency on others.

So if you are having trouble walking and you can't take care of the problem yourself, have a long talk with your doctor. Usually something can be done. The longer that you have been unable to walk, the more difficult the solution.

With arthritis, fatigue can cause a decrease in your desire to walk; this must be combatted. Or problems with the ball of the foot, the ankles, the knees, the hips, or the walking muscles can be responsible for the difficulty. It is partly a medical problem and partly a social one.

HOME TREATMENT

Be sure that the treatment for your arthritis is right. Are you taking your medication regularly? Do you need a change in medication? Could this be a side effect of a medication? Is your exercise program progressing smoothly?

Is a single joint causing the trouble? Could this joint be injected? Do you perhaps have a joint infection? Is this the time to consider surgery for that knee or hip? These and similar questions will help you decide on a strategy to get walking again.

A cane is the simplest aid to walking. It is usually held in the hand opposite an affected hip and on the most comfortable side for a bad knee. The usual C-handled cane is not really designed to be held easily, so you might prefer one with a functional grip handle. Some handles may need to be built up with tape to allow a good grip.

Crutches give somewhat more support but are more cumbersome. When you use crutches, your weight should not be on your armpits but on your arms. You may have to pad the grip or fit a knob to the crutch to get a good grip. The armpit is laced with fragile nerves and blood vessels and pressure there for very long can cause damage. If your grip is not too good, forearm platform crutches help you take the weight on the forearm. Bags can be attached to the crutch to allow you to carry small items—you just don't have enough hands for a purse or a package otherwise.

Walkers give stable support but are difficult to use for long distances. They are most useful about the house and while you're getting back on your feet after a flare-up or operation.

Don't forget the importance of correct footwear. If foot pain is limiting your walking, you will want to refer to some of the hints given in Pain in the Ball of the Foot **(S7)** and Heel Pain **(S8).**

Then there are gliders and wheelchairs. These are a subject in themselves. Good information is available from the Arthritis Foundation or the Arthritis Society, or from your physical therapist or occupational therapist. The goal, of course, is to keep you out of a wheelchair; each of the measures mentioned above helps you strengthen your body.

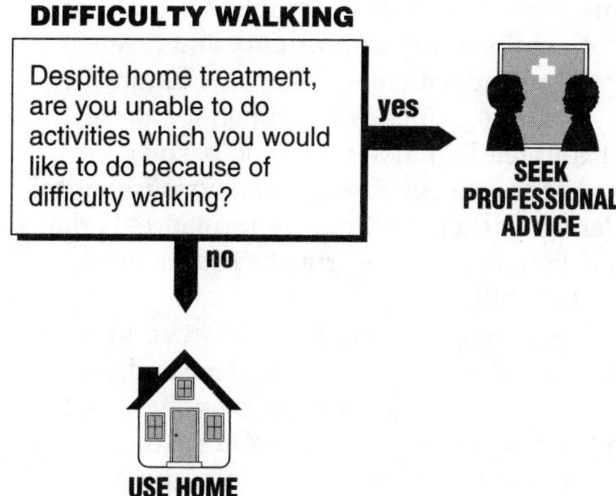

WHAT TO EXPECT FROM THE HEALTH PROFESSIONAL

The physical therapist will help you get started with appliances for walking assistance and will instruct you in exercises to strengthen your legs. The occupational therapist can help with additional adaptive devices. Social workers may assist in mobilizing community resources to help you. Your doctor will want to take a very serious look at your treatment program to ensure that all of the right things are being done.

SYMPTOM S32

32 Sexual Problems

Problems with sexual relationships occur much more often than would be suspected from the frequency of their discussion. Surprisingly, the patient is often not consciously aware of a sexual problem. Or the patient may be embarrassed to bring up the subject, especially an older patient who feels that sexual problems are not supposed to be an issue at certain ages. The doctor seldom asks specifically about sexual problems. Books either omit the subject or include a glib discussion about finding more comfortable sexual positions.

There is no single solution to these complex problems. There are as many different kinds of sexual needs and preferences as there are personalities. Trying to match some arbitrary definition of normal is exactly what you do not want to do. Instead, you should seek what is comfortable for you and your partner. Your own decisions will be determined by your background, your preferences before you had arthritis, the availability of a partner, and the needs and preferences of that partner. Problems can be discussed under three categories: frustration, manipulation, and guilt.

FRUSTRATION

This is the problem that comes first to mind, and the one that may be most easily managed. Basically, the frustrated person wants and needs sexual release, but cannot obtain it with sufficient frequency. The motive is there; the problem is one of opportunity and means. Perhaps the patient's self-image, diminished by arthritis, impedes the initiation of a sexual encounter. Perhaps there is no partner. Perhaps the process of sexual relations is painful. Perhaps disability limits performance. Perhaps a drug taken for the arthritis is decreasing sexual ability.

Self-image is critically important to sexual function. In this book, we've repeatedly stressed the dangers of perceiving yourself as a "victim" or an "invalid." You need confidence to face the challenges imposed by your arthritis. Sexual function can mirror your general opinion of yourself. The emotional aspects of sex are more important than the physical. Loneliness, depression, and isolation are more damaging than sexual abstinence. Sexual relationships can be a way of enhancing your self-image and the general level of your personal satisfaction.

From this viewpoint, you can avoid sexual failure even though technical difficulties with sexual performance persist. You can be sexually attractive. Attractiveness is related to caring, to careful listening, to respect for your partner. Dress attractively. Control your body weight. Groom carefully. The sexual solutions may well follow renewed respect for yourself.

The missing partner is a frequent and often overlooked problem. Sexual frequency in older individuals is strongly related to the availability of a sexual partner. Since women live considerably longer, on the average, than do men, the problem is often that of a widow, and is aggravated if the person is living alone with few social contacts. Sometimes sex is not a problem at all in this setting; if it is not, do not make it one. There is no rule that says there is no life after sex. If you do have a problem, masturbation is a possible answer.

Medically, this is an excellent means of physical release, but the guilt experienced by some people prevents it from being a perfect solution.

Seeking a partner is a neglected solution that can be thoroughly satisfactory at any age. The thrill of the September courtship is often as intense as that of young lovers, and many problems associated with arthritis are greatly helped by the presence of a partner.

If sexual activities are painful, there are a number of possible steps you can take. Keep in mind that prolonged foreplay increases vaginal lubrication and eases penetration, decreasing effort and pain. A vaginal lubricant, such as K-Y Jelly, may be used. Rheumatoid arthritis, in particular, often has vaginal dryness as one of its complications, so don't interpret lack of lubrication as sexual dysfunction. Better control of the arthritis will help, so discuss medications with your doctor. Anti-inflammatory medicine, taken two hours before intercourse, can help. Avoid painkillers since they often depress desire and sexual function. Urinate prior to intercourse. Take a warm bath if it helps you relax and loosen up. Use music to partially distract you from minor discomfort. Get comfortable in anticipation.

Position during intercourse can be varied, by trial and error, to find the most satisfactory. There is no single most satisfactory position. The standard advice is for the partner with arthritis to assume the more passive, usually underneath, role—but this does *not* consistently work. Sometimes one side or the other, male-inferior, male-superior, or posterior-entry positions work better. Some patients get a lot of benefit from using such simple devices as knee pads to protect sore knees or a pillow beneath the buttocks. Manual stimulation and oral stimulation can be less strenuous aspects of the love act.

Consider the best time of day to have sexual relations, particularly if you are bothered by fatigue in the afternoon or stiffness in the morning. For some, the middle of the day is most satisfactory. The more experimentation you feel comfortable with, the greater your chances of hitting the right combination. But don't force your emotional comfort; don't attempt sexual maneuvers that make you feel emotionally uncomfortable.

Disability can absolutely limit sexual activity, but this is extremely rare. Contractures of both hips in a female is the most frequent of such problems and may well be a signal to consider surgery.

Drugs are a frequently overlooked cause of sexual dysfunction. Alcohol, painkillers, sedatives, and tranquilizers all depress desire and ability, although in small doses each may act to facilitate relaxation. Drugs given to control a problem with the blood pressure pose a more direct problem; Aldomet and Ismelin, for example, very frequently impair male sexual function. Suspect almost any drug and talk with your doctor about it. If a drug is causing impotence, then the solution is simple. You just stop the drug or substitute a different drug.

MANIPULATION

This problem is major, frequent, and seldom recognized either by the manipulating partner or the one being manipulated. Here, one partner is using arthritis to avoid sexual encounters or to make the other feel bad about the imposition. This problem is rooted in the relationship, not in the sex itself.

Obesity has recently been identified as being, in some individuals, a mechanism to decrease sexual attractiveness and thus to avoid stresses related to sexual encounters.

Arthritis can, on occasion, be used in the same way. The sexual dysfunction in such cases will be out of proportion to the actual physical problem. This mechanism is similar to the classic "I've got a headache" technique for postponement of sexual activity. This is a big problem: The secondary gain (avoidance of sex) the patient gets from being disabled leads to therapeutic frustration—the patient doesn't really want to be well.

The same passive manipulation technique can be used in reverse by the nonarthritic partner. Here, sexual difficulties are interpreted as deliberate aggravation, even though the disability and problems are real. The partner without arthritis is trying to increase guilt and to decrease the self-image of the partner with arthritis—sort of a revenge tactic.

These problems are very hard to recognize and often harder to solve. The answer is, of course, for both partners to open up direct channels of communication and to negotiate, as adults, for the best solution: "It's not really the arthritis so much; I just really would like to have sex less often." "I get frustrated because of your arthritis, and I guess I've been pushing you on sex to try and get rid of my anger."

If such communication can develop, a negotiated solution is usually possible. The techniques of the previous section may be helpful. If the needs of the partners remain far apart, the entire relationship needs careful assessment. Marriage counselors or sexual counseling can help. But such problems usually were present before the arthritis, and such deep-rooted habit patterns are extremely difficult to change.

GUILT

The best sex relationships are free of guilt. This means greatly different things to different people; there can be no rigid rules. Many recent discussions of sex have been condemnations of old sexual taboos; sensual experiences previously considered deviant are now vigorously encouraged. This has generated a sort of reverse guilt in some. Now one can be guilty for not doing, while previously one was made to feel guilty for doing.

The sexual styles of different generations vary like shirt collars or skirt lengths. There is no single right answer, and the general rules fall before the particular instance. Some people feel awkward or undignified with certain sexual positions. Some find oral sex distasteful or experience prolonged guilt after masturbation. What is biologically equivalent may not be emotionally equivalent. Guilt over some sexual practice, guilt over nonperformance, guilt over infrequency, guilt over abstinence—all of these are detrimental. The practices with which you and your partner are most comfortable are the right ones. There is no harm. It is your sex life.

SYMPTOM S33

33 Problems with Employment

Winston Churchill used to follow a political and military strategy of "keeping all options open." This is the basic employment strategy for a person with significant arthritis.

PROBLEMS AND REALITIES

Let's look at some typical problems. A woman patient with recent onset of rheumatoid arthritis experiences fatigue, depression, and a problem with adjustment. Treatment has not yet been very helpful. She begins to work more slowly, misses some time, and her employer notes that her value to the company is decreasing. Her perception of failure on the job results in more depression, and the cycle continues until she either quits or gets fired.

A patient with Reiter's syndrome is unable to carry out work duties because of painful feet and ankles. Or advanced osteoarthritis of the knees causes a patient sufficient pain and disability to contemplate surgery—and lost time. Or a patient with inflamed finger joints from rheumatoid arthritis is advised not to work at an occupation that requires heavy use of the hands.

There are many such scenarios. Arthritis, defined broadly, causes more disability and more work time lost than any other set of human conditions.

Now let's look at the realities. That new rheumatoid arthritis patient will adjust to the problem and the disease will be controlled by medication. The Reiter's syndrome will subside as the particular flare-up ends. The contemplated knee surgery will restore function and decrease pain for the immobile patient with osteoarthritis. The inflamed finger joints, over months, will become much better, and that patient will accept a better-paying job in the accounting department. Each of these patients will become employable again and each will do a good job.

Work is a very positive thing. It promotes independence, self-fulfillment, and problem-solving skills. It provides money, which decreases one set of worries. It encourages active social interaction with other people. We like our patients to go on working despite their arthritis and to return to work if they have to stop temporarily. The pain message and your common sense will tell you what you can do.

THE BAD NEWS AND THE GOOD NEWS

Unfortunately, there is a negative side to the employment question, and it reflects poorly on our society. The patient with arthritis has been neglected by the politician and by the social planner. Sick leave, medical insurance, unemployment programs, and disability awards are not designed for the intermediate term of six to twelve months, and they often discriminate against musculoskeletal disability. The Americans with Disabilities Act is beginning, however, to make a positive contribution.

Sometimes if you return to work from disability status, you lose the right to go back on it if things don't work out. What a crazy system! Sometimes an employer will discriminate, in spite of antidiscrimination laws, against patients with arthritis, fearing that their productivity will be lower and their sick time more frequent.

Political lobbies for the disabled have concentrated on the paraplegic patient and the patient with spinal cord injury instead of the much more common problem of arthritis. Definitions of "physically handicapped" are often narrow, excluding patients with arthritis. The situation is lamentably inflexible. Our view is that disability arrangements are not required for the arthritis patient too often, but when they are needed it is a gross injustice for them to be difficult to obtain. Your support of the Arthritis Foundation or Arthritis Society, nationally and locally, can help improve this situation.

Now the better news. Social solutions for disability can be found. Be persistent with public officials and insurance companies. It helps if you have a doctor or social worker who knows the local situation well. Several letters from the doctor may be needed. Highly placed officials of some insurance plans have told me that first claims for disability payment are often automatically rejected by the computer, but that follow-up requests are then evaluated on their merits. So be persistent.

HOW TO HELP YOURSELF

Then there is your part. As always, you play the biggest role in solving your problems. The hints in the previous problem discussions will help. Your expectations must be both positive and realistic. And you must be determined.

Figure out your prognosis. Check the questionnaire in Appendix A to find out how bad your arthritis is; pay particular attention to your "daily function" score. Read the general prognosis for your kind of arthritis in Part I. And remember that after a year or so of arthritis you can predict the future pretty well by analyzing the past; you are unlikely to get any brand-new problems after that period.

Is your present job right for you? Retraining or job transfer is best accomplished if there isn't any rush and if you are employed at the time of inquiry. Wait for the right opening and transfer into it. If you anticipate slowly increasing difficulty with a particular activity, make plans to avoid that activity.

The patient with significant arthritis often has major advantages over people with other handicaps. Most importantly, the brain usually works fine. So do the heart and the lungs. The person beneath the outward infirmity is well equipped to adjust to problems with pain or mobility.

The adjustment is not easy and it would be nice if the system were more hassle-free, but employment problems can be solved. Productive life despite arthritis is the goal, and it can be achieved.

PART IV

Appendixes

A. *Rate Your Arthritis*

B. *Information Sources*

APPENDIX A

Rate Your Arthritis

This Arthritis Status Test is used by arthritis centers to evaluate the status of their patients. You can score your own arthritis, and you can follow your own progress over time. For reference, compare your scores with those of patients at the Stanford Arthritis Center, provided in the "How to Interpret Your Score" section.

The Arthritis Status Test

Mark lightly with a pencil (you will want to use this test again) the one response that best describes your abilities.

The Arthritis Status Test

	Without difficulty	*With difficulty*	*With help from another*	*Unable to do at all*
Daily Function				
1. Dressing: Can you get your clothes, dress yourself, shampoo your hair . . . ?	______ 0	______ 1	______ 2	______ 3
2. Standing up: Are you able to stand up from a straight chair without using your arms to push off . . . ?	______ 0	______ 1	______ 2	______ 3

	Without difficulty	*With difficulty*	*With help from another*	*Unable to do at all*
Daily Function				
3. Eating: Can you cut your meat and lift a cup to your mouth . . . ?	0	1	2	3
4. Walking: Can you walk outdoors on flat ground . . . ?	0	1	2	3
5. Hygiene: Can you wash and dry your entire body, turn faucets, and get on and off the toilet . . . ?	0	1	2	3
6. Reach: Can you reach up to and get down a seven-pound (3 kg) object that is above your head . . . ?	0	1	2	3
7. Grip: Can you open jars that have been previously opened . . . ?	0	1	2	3
8. Activity: Can you drive a car or run errands and shop . . . ?	0	1	2	3
Pain and Discomfort				
1. Severity: How would you describe the pain from your arthritis over the past week?	0/None	1/Mild	2/Moderate	3/Severe
2. Trend: How has the severity of the pain changed over the past week?	0/No pain	1/Better	2/The same	3/Worse

That's the test. Now, put the numbers (0, 1, 2, 3) corresponding to your answers in the appropriate spaces of the first column of the Arthritis Rating Sheet that follows. The other columns are for repeating the test in the future; we recommend every six months. You must have answered all of the questions to have a valid score.

The Arthritis Rating Sheet

Date Rated	______	______	______	______	______	______
Daily Function						
1. Dressing	______	______	______	______	______	______
2. Standing up	______	______	______	______	______	______
3. Eating	______	______	______	______	______	______
4. Walking	______	______	______	______	______	______
5. Hygiene	______	______	______	______	______	______
6. Reach	______	______	______	______	______	______
7. Grip	______	______	______	______	______	______
8. Activity	______	______	______	______	______	______
Function points (Add 1 through 8)	______	______	______	______	______	______
Pain and Discomfort						
1. Severity	______	______	______	______	______	______
2. Trend	______	______	______	______	______	______
Pain points (Add 1 and 2)	______	______	______	______	______	______

How to Interpret Your Score

This status test has been used with over 2,000 patients with rheumatoid arthritis (RA) evaluated by the Stanford Arthritis Center. Most of these persons have had arthritis for five to ten years and have worse arthritis than the typical patient. You can compare your score with the figures below, which show the percentage of patients with different numbers of points.

Daily Function Points

Points	*Rating*	*Percent of RA patients*
0–4	Normal	36
5–12	Adequate	47
13–20	Impaired	16
21–24	Disabled	1

Pain and Discomfort Points

Points	*Rating*	*Percent of RA patients*
0	None	2
1–2	Mild	8
3–4	Moderate	64
5–6	Severe	26

Repeat your score every six months and date and record the results. You will be able to measure your improvement. If your scores are getting worse, it may be time to talk with your doctor about changing your treatment program.

APPENDIX B

Information Sources

Reading List

The following materials provide additional discussions of the topics in this book. I believe them to be basically sound and of potential value for the patient with arthritis.

Recommended Books About Arthritis and Rheumatism

Arthritis Foundation. *Understanding Arthritis,* Irving Kushner, M.D., editor. New York: Scribner's, 1984.

Fransen, Jenny and I. John Russell. *The Fibromyalgia Help Book.* St. Paul, Minn.: Smith House Press, 1996.

Fries, James F., M.D. *Living Well.* Reading, Mass.: Perseus, 1999.

Fries, James F., M.D. and Lawrence M. Crapo. *Vitality and Aging.* San Francisco: W. H. Freeman, 1981.

Lane, Nancy, M.D. *The Osteoporosis Book: A Guide for Patients and Their Families.* New York: Oxford Univeristy Press, 1999.

Lorig, Kate, R.N., Dr.P.H. and James F. Fries, M.D. *The Arthritis Helpbook,* 5th ed. Reading, Mass.: Perseus, 1999.

Moskowitz, Roland W., M.D. and Marie R. Haug, Ph.D. *Arthritis and the Elderly.* New York: Springer Publishing Company, 1986.

Schlotzhauer, Tammil, M.D. and James L. McGuire, M.D. *Living with Rheumatoid Arthritis.* Baltimore: Johns Hopkins University Press, 1993.

Swezey, Robert L., M.D. and Annette M. Swezey. *Good News for Bad Backs.* Santa Monica, Cal.: Cequal, 1994.

Vickery, Donald M., M.D. and James F. Fries, M.D. *Take Care of Yourself,* 6th ed. Reading, Mass.: Perseus, 1996.

Not Recommended

I believe these books to be oversimplified or misleading, sometimes dangerously so. They are given by title only.

There Is a Cure for Arthritis

Arthritis Can Be Cured

A Doctor's Proven New Home Cure for Arthritis

The Arthritic's Cookbook

New Hope for the Arthritic

Arthritis and Folk Medicine

Your Aching Back and What You Can Do About It

Arthritis, Nutrition, and Natural Therapy

Arthritis and Common Sense

Pamphlets Available from the Arthritis Foundation

Excellent pamphlets are available through your local chapter of the Arthritis Foundation or from the national Arthritis Foundation office, or from the Arthritis Society in Canada. Usually there is no charge for single copies; there is often a nominal charge for multiple copies to cover printing costs. Titles change; you should consult your local chapter for presently available materials. Here are two good ones.

Arthritis: The Basic Facts. 28 pages.

Self-help Manual for Arthritis Patients. 124 pages. Excellent.

Arthritis Organizations Around the World

The Arthritis Foundation in the United States, New Zealand, and Australia and the Arthritis Society in Canada are truly marvelous institutions. They sponsor programs in public education and professional education, support young professionals establishing research careers in arthritis, and provide direct support for research activities. They lead the fight for increased government programs of research and service in the U.S.

The Arthritis Foundation in the U.S. consists of a national office and local chapters around the country. You will usually want to contact the local chapter, which can advise you of doctors and clinics in your area, provide instructional materials, and occasionally help with financial problems. There may be a schedule of activities you can attend. Or you might want to volunteer your efforts in support of the chapter.

Look in the phone book under Arthritis Foundation or call 1-800-283-7800 for toll-free information in the United States. The address of the national office is:

The Arthritis Foundation
1314 Spring Street, N.W.
Atlanta, GA 30309

Organizations like the Arthritis Foundation also provide services in New Zealand, Australia, and Canada, as well as many other countries.

ARTHRITIS FOUNDATION OF NEW ZEALAND
P.O. Box 10-020
Wellington
Telephone: (04) 721-427

ARTHRITIS FOUNDATION OF AUSTRALIA
P.O. Box 121
Sydney NSW 2001
Telephone: (02) 221-2456

ARTHRITIS SOCIETY OF CANADA
250 Bloor Street East, Suite 401
Toronto, Ontario M4W 3P2
Telephone: (416) 967-1414

INDEX

Entries in **boldface** indicate the pages where you can find the most information on each subject. For common medical problems, these are usually the pages with decision charts and advice on home treatment and when to see a doctor.